The Memory Program

How to Prevent Memory Loss and Enhance Memory Power

D. P. Devanand, M.D.

D0711808

John Wiley & Sons, Inc.

New York • Chichester • Weinheim • Brisbane • Singapore • Toronto

In my father's memory

Copyright © 2001 by D. P. Devanand. All rights reserved

Published by John Wiley & Sons, Inc.
Published simultaneously in Canada

This publication is designed to provide accurate and authoritative information in regard to the subject matter covered. It is sold with the understanding that the publisher is not engaged in rendering professional services. If professional advice or other expert assistance is required, the services of a competent professional person should be sought.

This publication is the product of the author's own work done on his own time, and does not represent the views of either the New York State Psychiatric Institute or Columbia University. Any errors in fact or judgment are exclusively the author's own.

Library of Congress Cataloging-in-Publication Data:
Devanand, D. P.
 The memory program : how to prevent memory loss and enhance memory power /
D.P. Devanand
  p. cm.
 Includes bibliographical references and index.
 ISBN 0-471-39833-0 (pbk.)
 1. Memory disorders–Prevention. 2. Memory. I. Title
RC394.M46 D483 2001
616.8′4–dc21
                     00-053409

Printed in the United States of America

10 9 8 7 6 5 4 3 2 1

CONTENTS

PREFACE

As the population ages, there is growing concern about mild memory loss and how to prevent it. Many people fear losing their memory, some are uncertain about the boundaries between normal aging and pathologic memory loss, and others have questions about which preventive and treatment measures are safe and really work. These questions have gained added momentum because a plethora of exciting new preventive strategies and treatments have been developed for memory loss: from alternative medications like ginkgo biloba to dietary supplements like vitamin E to cholinesterase inhibitors like donepezil (Aricept), rivastigmine (Exelon), and galantamine (Reminyl) that are approved by the Food and Drug Administration (FDA) to treat Alzheimer's disease.

As a practicing physician and researcher, I have been immersed in academic pursuits for the last sixteen years, publishing two books and over 130 papers, supported by a number of clinical research grants, mainly from the National Institutes of Health. But over time, as I began to wonder about how much of this new knowledge actually percolates down to the general public, the outline for this book began to take shape in my mind. After researching a large number of books that are available to the general public, I discovered that there wasn't a single source that provided comprehensive information about memory loss and how to prevent and treat it, utilizing a memory program that could be tailor-made for each individual. Translating the available medical and scientific evidence into information that the average person can use in his or her daily life has been my goal in writing this book.

This book describes the current state of knowledge about memory loss due to the aging process, provides specific guidelines to prevent memory loss, and reviews established and breakthrough treatments for memory loss. I rely on the scientific evidence, buttressed by my clinical experience, in developing each element of the

Memory Program that the reader can utilize on a day-to-day basis. When pertinent, I describe the stories of interesting patients (identities disguised) as well as other anecdotes to illustrate the rationale behind specific components of the Memory Program.

This book is meant for people who have a normal memory and wish to prevent memory loss as they grow older, as well as for people (including perhaps your parents and other loved ones) who already suffer from mild memory loss and wish to prevent further decline. This book is not meant for people with severe memory loss or dementia, for which other books are readily available.

After the introduction, the book is divided into five parts. In the first part, The Basics of Memory, you will learn how to evaluate your memory using simple tests, how memory works in the brain, and how aging affects this process. In the second part, Start the Memory Program, the various elements in the Memory Program are introduced, and a diet and exercise plan is described. This section ends with a detailed description of specific memory training techniques. In the third part, Prevent and Treat Common Causes of Memory Loss, the focus is on depression, alcohol abuse, hormonal and nutritional problems, and a number of other reversible factors that commonly cause memory loss. This is an important part of the book, because having a reversible cause that is left undiagnosed and untreated could result in a tragedy. In the penultimate section, Medications That Prevent and Treat Memory Loss, alternative (usually natural substances), over-the-counter, and prescription medications to treat memory loss are comprehensively reviewed, both from a research and clinical perspective. This provides a stepping-stone to the final part, Putting It All Together, where the Memory Program is described in great detail, utilizing all the elements that have been developed in earlier chapters. The generic memory program is followed by a section that individualizes the program for people in specific categories, for example, women who are forty to fifty-nine years old with no memory loss, men who are sixty years or older with mild memory loss, etc.

A word of caution. The ideal study to evaluate a long-term strategy to prevent memory loss due to the aging process would systematically evaluate young or middle-aged people and then institute long-term preventive interventions (such as diet, exercise, memory training, or medications) with regular follow-up and assessment over a period of thirty to fifty years. There has been no such study, partly because practical problems make such a long-term project very difficult to execute, and partly because the issue of memory loss has gained prominence only in recent years. Nonetheless, the evidence from a variety of short-term to intermediate-term (a few months to a few years) studies is strong enough to provide a solid foundation to develop and implement a comprehensive program to prevent memory loss due to the aging process.

One final issue to consider is called the practice effect. When you first try to complete neuropsychological tests, which include the tests of memory that you will take in the first chapter, some parts seem difficult. The next time you do the same tests, you are likely to perform better, even on those tests that seemed hard to do the first time. This is the practice effect, which means that repeated testing results in superior performance because the brain automatically (even without conscious learning) begins to figure out how best to do the test. In people with little to no memory loss, the practice effect can last for many months after only a single testing session. Therefore, if test performance is compared before and after treatment for memory loss, there will often be some improvement due to the practice effect. If, however, active treatment (medication or diet alteration or memory training or any other intervention) is compared to placebo, subtracting the change on placebo (sugar pill) from the change on active treatment gives us the real effect. This would take into account the practice effect, which is assumed to be equal in people on active treatment and people on placebo. In other words, it is easy to show that a treatment intervention leads to improved memory by retesting the subject, but the only sound way to show that this improvement is not caused by the practice effect is to conduct a placebo-controlled study. This issue is critical in evaluating the merits of any of the treatments described in this book, or any other information that you may come across in the media about the treatment of memory loss.

Despite these reservations, the available evidence provides considerable room for optimism. I suggest that you begin, and then maintain, the Memory Program to prevent memory loss, and to directly tackle mild memory loss if it has already begun to affect your life. Over an extended period of time, you are likely to look back with satisfaction at the results that you have achieved.

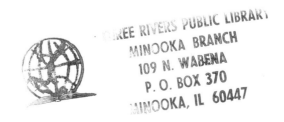

ACKNOWLEDGMENTS

W HEN I WAS TRAINING in the early 1980s at Yale, Dr. Craig Nelson helped me write and publish a paper on the interface between memory loss and depression. He was an outstanding mentor and helped propel me in the direction of studying and treating memory disorders, which I have been doing for the last sixteen years. While Dr. Nelson remained at Yale, I moved to the medical center at Columbia University, where I have stayed ever since. At Columbia, many teachers, professional colleagues, and students, too numerous to name individually, have helped shape my thinking, clinical expertise, and research ideas and projects in dealing with the problems of memory loss due to the aging process and related disorders. This thriving clinical-cum-research environment is likely to continue well into the future, and I owe all the individuals involved a great debt. In particular, I would like to thank all my patients and their families, from whom I have learned a great deal. I believe I was able to help them a little in their struggle against memory loss, and I drew on this experience in formulating the Memory Program that is central to this book.

My literary agent, Lynn Franklin, patiently kept me on track from the inception of the book proposal to the completion of this book. Her critical comments and advice helped me keep concepts clear and simple for the reader. Tom Miller at John Wiley provided incisive editorial comments that helped make this an informative yet practical book for people who wish to learn about memory loss and how to prevent and treat it.

INTRODUCTION

David's Story

In the spring of 1988, a short, overweight corporate executive wearing a three-piece suit walked into my office at the Columbia University Memory Disorders Center. David Finestone* was forty-nine years old. He sat stiffly, with his hands clasped to the armrests of his chair.

"Doctor, I think I'm getting Alzheimer's disease," he announced, sweating visibly.

I listened carefully to his story, wondering how I could help him. He had recently begun having difficulty remembering names. This symptom, which he had never experienced before in his life, had started barely three months earlier. He described an episode when he forgot the name of an important client and had trouble introducing this client by name to a colleague. David was afraid that if his memory lapses continued, they could lead to his being laid off in the corporate downsizing frenzy that prevailed at that time. For obvious reasons, he had not spoken about this issue to anyone at work and hadn't even discussed it with his wife. He had begun to lose his self-confidence, because this was the first time that he had ever doubted his own intellectual capabilities. He was used to facing obstacles head-on and overcoming them, and he told me that he would do whatever was needed to solve his memory problem, even if it meant making personal sacrifices. I considered his fighting spirit and willingness to change to be very good signs, and reassured him that I would do everything possible to get to the root of his problem.

The symptom of difficulty in remembering names tends to develop gradually in many middle-aged people, but David was

---

*Not his real name; all names and identifying features of patients are completely disguised in this book.

1

insistent that his lapses had begun abruptly. I put him through a battery of tests, which included a complete medical, neurological, and
psychiatric evaluation, several blood tests to look for nutritional and
hormonal causes of memory loss, an MRI (magnetic resonance imaging) scan to evaluate brain structure, and a SPECT (single photon
emission computerized tomography) scan to assess blood flow in different brain regions. This extensive workup revealed an abnormality
on the SPECT scan: a small decrease in blood flow in the left temporal lobe, the critical region that includes the hippocampus, the
main seat of memory in the brain. Detailed neuropsychological testing, which involved a variety of paper and pencil tests, confirmed a
deficit in memory for names. Otherwise, his memory and intellectual
performance were in the normal range.

A history of an abrupt onset of memory loss often points to a
stroke that is caused by decreased blood supply. The neuropsychological test results and SPECT findings seemed to confirm this possibility. I concluded that a localized deficit in blood flow, probably a
"ministroke," had affected a small part of the temporal lobe that controls memory for names. A ministroke means that the cutoff in blood
supply affects such a small portion of brain tissue that usually no
symptoms are reported when the stroke occurs, as was the case with
David Finestone. Only later had he begun to notice memory loss. The
radiologist had read his MRI scan as normal, but MRI technology was
not, and still is not, capable of picking up very small strokes less than
2 mm (one-tenth of an inch) in size. While I couldn't absolutely rule
out very early Alzheimer's disease—a condition in which memory
deficits are widespread and not restricted to forgetting names—this
diagnosis seemed very unlikely. I discussed the results in detail with
David, and told him that he was lucky he hadn't yet had a clinical
stroke, the cause of his father's untimely death. I reassured him that
there was a high probability his symptom could indeed be prevented
from worsening, if not fully reversed. He let out an audible sigh of
relief and listened carefully to my advice.

I suggested that he change his lifestyle, both for general health
reasons and to prevent the risk of stroke and further memory loss.
He followed through on my instruction to decrease the intake of saturated fats in his diet, which in his case included red meat and milk
products, especially pizza, which he had two to three times a week.
He started eating more fresh fruit and green vegetables, and began
a regular exercise regimen. He also acted on my recommendation to
take an aspirin a day to reduce the risk of future strokes, and 800 units
daily of vitamin E for its antioxidant properties, which can delay both

the aging process and memory loss. He returned to see me every six months for the next two years, and neuropsychological testing showed a gradual improvement in his memory for names. During this period, he lost twenty pounds and became more energetic and productive— so much so that he not only kept his job but was also promoted to general manager of his division. He was delighted, and so was I. David Finestone was now convinced that his occasional difficulty in remembering names was not the first sign of Alzheimer's disease, and we both agreed that he didn't need to consult me anymore.

Frieda's Story

Later that year, Frieda Kohlberg, a seventy-four-year-old woman who had survived the Holocaust, was brought in by her husband, who felt that his wife's razor-sharp mind was beginning to fail. She had forgotten to shut off the electric stove on one occasion and had seemed a little confused at a friend's house. At other times, she remained mentally sharp and continued to read a book every week.

Tall and stately, Mrs. Kohlberg walked into my office in a well-tailored blue serge dress, her curly blond hair perfectly set for the occasion. She sat down, announced that she did not have a memory problem, and to prove it, spontaneously began to recite the latest items in the news without the slightest difficulty. On a brief memory test, she could remember two out of three unrelated nouns (bus, door, rose) after a delay of five minutes. This slight deficit is not uncommon in people of her age but can sometimes be an early sign of dementia. (Dementia is a broad diagnosis that includes several brain diseases, including Alzheimer's, which is the cause of 60 to 70 percent of all cases of dementia and typically produces severe memory loss and decline with eventual inability to carry out daily functions and activities.) Since I wasn't entirely sure about where Mrs. Kohlberg stood along the spectrum of memory loss, I ordered several blood tests to look for possible causes like thyroid or vitamin deficiencies. These tests, as well as MRI and SPECT scans of the brain, were completely normal. Neuropsychological testing confirmed slight impairment in recent memory but no other intellectual deficits. In fact, her IQ score was 154—in the genius range. My neuropsychologist colleagues and I put our heads together to try to resolve these conflicting results. On the one hand, her slight deficit in recent memory was within the lower limit of the "normal" range for people of her age. On the other hand, someone with her high

IQ should have been able to ace the tests, including the memory component, without the slightest difficulty. When the frontline mechanism for memory fails, highly intelligent people like Mrs. Kohlberg are capable of bringing into play a number of alternate brain circuits to make up for the deficit, and this can deceive the doctor into thinking that there is no risk of dementia. I was afraid that her test results showed this had begun to happen. I also gave extra weight to her husband's report that she had become confused at a friend's house.

To the best of my ability, I conveyed the ambiguity of the test results to Frieda Kohlberg and her husband.

"I'm not at all worried about my memory. I feel fine, there's nothing wrong with my head. I'm not a crazy person," she insisted. "So I don't see why I need to come back anymore."

Her reaction was not a good sign, because denial of memory loss when it actually exists often indicates that the patient is crossing the bridge from mild memory loss to early Alzheimer's disease. Her husband remained concerned and convinced her to come back for follow-up testing every six months. To my dismay, and her husband's, her memory steadily worsened over the next two years until she met clinical diagnostic criteria for Alzheimer's disease. At that time, there were no worthwhile treatment options for this dreaded illness, and eventually she needed round-the-clock nursing care at home. Her husband was emphatic that she never be placed in an institution of any type, and that he himself would do everything possible to keep her at home until the very end, no matter what toll it took on his own life. I decided to support his decision, even though I usually advise family members to consider reasonable alternative living situations if the burden of caring for a patient with advanced dementia becomes overwhelming.

Mild Memory Loss: What Does It Mean?

I learned a lot from these two patients of mine. They highlight the difficulty in interpreting the meaning of mild memory loss that usually develops as you grow older. Sometimes it is benign and does not progress, but at other times it is the first sign of dementia. These clinical experiences led me to study early diagnostic markers for Alzheimer's disease in people with mild memory loss. But after conducting extensive research funded by the National Institutes of Health, I still have more questions than answers. Although several exciting new findings have emerged from this research and those of other investigators, the fundamental breakthrough still lies in the future. Nonetheless, research's increased focus on dementia—and memory loss more broadly—has vastly expanded our knowledge base and has helped to develop effective preventive strategies and treatments for memory loss. This is truly a sea change from barely a decade ago, when the symptom of memory loss usually led to the view that "senility" had set in and could not be stopped. I wish that some of these new treatments had been available for Frieda Kohlberg when she developed memory loss, because they could have slowed down the rapid progression of her terrible illness.

David Finestone and Frieda Kohlberg were unusual patients for me to see in 1988. At that time, most patients who came to our Memory Disorders Center already had moderate to advanced dementia, most commonly Alzheimer's disease. But during the 1990s, the number of middle-aged and elderly people who had mild memory complaints and deficits literally ballooned. They asked me the same questions with almost alarming regularity:

- I have mild memory loss. Is that normal or abnormal for my age?
- If my memory loss is abnormal, does that mean I am getting Alzheimer's disease?
- If my memory worsens, how can I prevent my own personality, my "self," from being destroyed?

There Are New Preventive and Treatment Strategies

In the new millennium, these fears have been turned on their head with discoveries of new preventive strategies and a whole range of treatments for memory loss. I now face a brand-new set of questions that ask which preventive measures should be taken and which treatments for memory loss are safe and really work. As a practicing physician and an active researcher in the field of memory disorders, in writing this book I relied on the available medical and scientific information, buttressed by my own clinical experience, to explain how memory works and then describe the best methods to prevent and treat memory loss.

The Memory Program is intended to help two categories of people:

1. The large number of middle-aged people, mainly baby boomers, who currently have a normal memory and wish to preserve their memory as they grow older.
2. The smaller number of people with mild memory loss, middle-aged and older, who would like to reverse the process or at least prevent further decline in their memory.

You Can Prevent Memory Loss Now

The baby boom generation has an overriding concern—even obsession—with quality-of-life issues. They are doing everything possible to prevent the aging process, including memory loss, from taking hold of their lives. To help maintain peak physical and mental function, a balanced diet and a fitness program have become the dual mantra for tens of millions. And as the baby boomers age, they will dwell even more on maintaining optimal physical and mental health.

By the year 2025, over eighty million baby boomers will have entered the zone of Social Security and Medicare, and there will be two people over sixty-five for every teenager in the United States. As the population ages, awareness about the importance of living well and not just living longer has led to growing concern about several conditions that were widely believed to be "subclinical" and hence unimportant. These include mild symptoms of arthritis, depression, and memory loss, which are extremely common in the general population. Community surveys show that mild memory loss is present in 1 to 10 percent of people between the ages of forty-five and sixty-five, and in 10 to 40 percent among those sixty-five to eighty-five years of age. Nearly half the middle-aged and elderly people living in the United States worry about their memory, and objective testing has confirmed that subtle memory loss is indeed widespread. Memory is the mental function that declines the most rapidly as we grow older, and this huge public health problem will mushroom in the decades to come.

Do You Need the Memory Program?

If you have a reversible cause of memory loss that can be recognized and treated effectively, such as depression or vitamin deficiency or hormonal abnormality, a "cure" is possible. But for the more common condition of age-related memory loss, where there is no clear-cut reversible cause, you need many strategies, including general health measures (diet, exercise, memory training, and nutritional supplements) and new medications (natural/alternative, over-the-counter, and prescription). All these components are integral parts of the Memory Program developed in this book, which you can tailor to your individual needs. In particular, you should recognize that there is no magic pill, no magic bullet, that can turn you into a memory superwoman or superman. To help preserve and even improve your memory, a comprehensive, multifaceted program is the right solution.

If you are frightened about losing your memory, you should read *The Memory Program*. And even if you have a normal memory, you should seriously consider a promemory program because a decline in memory is likely during the natural process of aging. Nearly everyone above the age of forty can benefit from reading this book, with the exception of people with severe memory loss or dementia, for whom other books are readily available.

The book is divided into the following sections:

1. A description of normal aging and memory processes that includes tests for you to determine whether your memory is normal or abnormal;
2. Proactive general health measures to prevent memory loss: diet, physical exercise, and memory training techniques;
3. Identification and treatment of common, usually reversible, causes of memory loss;
4. A careful analysis of alternative, over-the-counter, and prescription medications to prevent and treat memory loss;
5. A final major section that pulls all this information together into a comprehensive memory program tailored for each of you, and touches on future directions in memory loss research.

I suggest that you read this book from beginning to end without skipping chapters, because some of the material later in the book builds on information presented in earlier chapters. But if you have a scientific or medical background and already know a great deal about the nature of memory loss and the available prevention and treatment strategies, you should feel free to go directly to the chapters that address your specific concerns.

Take a Proactive Approach

The main premise of this book is that preventing and treating memory loss requires active intervention, not a passive approach. Just as advances in technology double the performance of computers every twelve to eighteen months, biomedical research is literally doubling our medical knowledge base every few years. With the knowledge that we now have (which is reviewed comprehensively in this book), and the new advances made every day, we're headed toward a complete understanding of memory loss due to the aging process—and eventually a cure.

PART ONE

The Basics of Memory

CHAPTER 1

Evaluate Your Memory

A good storyteller is a person who has a good memory,
and hopes other people haven't.
—IRVIN S. COBB, AMERICAN HUMORIST

Woody Allen once said that the brain was his second favorite organ. While the brain may indeed be the number two choice for many of us, it is by far our most important organ, and memory is one of its most critical functions.

In this part of the book, you will learn how to assess your memory and determine whether it is normal or abnormal. You will also learn about the basic processes underlying memory formation and retrieval in the brain, and how aging affects these processes. This information will help you fully understand the reasoning behind the different elements in the Memory Program.

Everyone Forgets

Some of us forget names; others cannot recall places they've been to before. Our ability to associate names, faces, and places in the context of time helps us to reinforce our memories. Lost memories that suddenly resurface indicate that our brains store much more information than we are aware of in everyday life. Sigmund Freud was convinced that the root cause of "forgetting" is an unconscious conflict that creates a mental block when we consciously try to remember.

11

While this theory may apply to some people, as we grow older there is a different type of memory loss that affects most of us. This memory loss is a direct result of the aging process.

Benign versus Malignant Memory Loss

In the 1960s, V. A. Kral, a Canadian physician, coined the term "benign senescent forgetfulness" to describe the mild memory loss that he observed in older people, which he distinguished from the more malignant memory loss that is an early sign of dementia. Kral's terminology has been replaced by "age-associated memory impairment" (AAMI) and "age-related cognitive decline" (ARCD). *Cognition* is a word used to describe a wide range of intellectual functions, including memory. The term "mild cognitive impairment" (MCI) defines a broad group of people who have cognitive deficits and fall between the categories of "normal" and "dementia." Although the original "benign senescent forgetfulness" is rapidly disappearing from the field, it is still useful to recognize that memory loss during aging is often "benign," because it does not worsen markedly over time, especially if sound preventive measures are employed. My patient David Finestone was a case in point: he adopted a systematic program that improved his memory and overall level of functioning.

Forgetting Names

I have always tended to forget the names of people when I am introduced to them for the first time. I am sure that many of the people I met were convinced that I forgot their names because I didn't really care one way or another. In some cases this was true. But even when I do make a conscious effort to remember a name, I often cannot retain it unless it is repeated back to me. Even more embarrassing is when I meet someone who crossed my path some months or years ago and I discover that I am absolutely clueless about that person's name. I wouldn't be surprised if some of you have had similar experiences, though hopefully not as often as I've had.

Before I started studying memory loss, I preferred to forget this personal flaw. However, at the back of my mind was the memory of how my mother used to constantly joke about my late father's inability to remember names. I grew up in Calcutta, India, and my father would regularly call Mr. Chatterjee by the name of Mr. Banerjee while

Mr. Ghosh became Mr. Das. My father gave a few unfortunate souls four or five names on different occasions. In striking contrast, my mother always had a razor sharp recall for names. This facility only doubled her amusement at my father's gaffes, which often led to his laughing at himself. But observing these patterns in my family led me to wonder: is the ability to recall names mainly genetic? If so, I would have a great excuse for my shoddy recall of names, though blaming my father's genes for this deficit does sound like a lame excuse.

Forgetting names is a widespread, almost universal, phenomenon. Some of you may agree with my self-serving explanation that there is a strong genetic component. However, forgetting names is not in itself a clinical syndrome, and few researchers have exerted much time or energy to get to the root of this problem, genetic or otherwise. There has been one remarkable exception: Albert DaMasio, a neurologist who is a giant in his field.

The Tip-of-the-Tongue Phenomenon

In a compelling paper published in the journal *Nature,* DaMasio and his colleagues showed that the areas of the brain that encode and store memories of proper nouns are distinct from those responsible for other kinds of nouns, even though these regions are physically very close to one another and are near the hippocampus, which forms part of the temporal lobe in the brain. His work has taught us a great deal about how different elements of memory are stored and helps explain the tip-of-the-tongue phenomenon. If memories for different types of words are stored in different groups of nerve cells, these nerve cells need to communicate with one another to produce a composite memory of the entire object or person that is rich in detail. If this communication does not occur, you may recall one element of the memory but not another, and the missing component remains on the tip of the tongue. This process of retrieval is not entirely conscious, because the "missing link" may suddenly resurface when your mind is preoccupied with something else, which somehow gives the nerve cells a better opportunity to communicate.

Symptoms of Memory Loss

Many other symptoms of memory loss are not as benign as forgetting names and are listed on the following page. If you (or someone close to you) have signs of severe memory loss, or if you've developed functional changes associated with memory loss, you should get your symptoms investigated by a doctor. The most important warning sign is a clear-cut *worsening* in memory compared to how you were a few months or years ago.

Early, Usually Benign, Signs of Memory Loss
- Forgetting names
- Forgetting a few items on a shopping list
- Misplacing keys, wallets, handbags
- Forgetting to turn off the stove once
- Losing your way in a giant mall
- Not recognizing someone you met a long time ago

Signs of Severe Memory Loss
- Getting lost in a familiar place
- Losing your way when driving a familiar route
- Forgetting important appointments repeatedly
- Forgetting to turn off the stove on several occasions
- Repeating the same questions over and over again
- Difficulty in understanding words or in speaking fluently
- Not knowing the date or time

Functional Changes Associated with Severe Memory Loss
- Problems at work; coworkers say that your poor memory is causing too many mistakes
- Making many errors in balancing a checkbook or writing checks
- Difficulty in naming common objects or finding words
- Apathy, irritability, and other personality changes accompanying memory loss

Seeing Your Doctor for Memory Loss

Any one of the following categories of professionals can evaluate memory loss:

- **PRIMARY CARE PHYSICIANS** (internists, family practitioners) can identify the medical causes of memory loss (e.g., hormonal abnormality or medication toxicity), but they often miss the early signs of subtle to mild memory loss because most are not very skilled at testing for it.

- **NEUROLOGISTS** are physicians trained in the diagnosis and evaluation of neurological disorders such as stroke and multiple sclerosis. They are generally good at identifying early signs of memory loss. However, only some neurologists have developed expertise in diagnosing and treating memory disorders.
- **PSYCHIATRISTS** have a medical degree and specialize in the treatment of mental disorders. They are excellent at identifying causes such as depression underlying memory loss. However, like most neurologists, most psychiatrists are not skilled at diagnosing and treating memory disorders.
- **NEUROPSYCHOLOGISTS** have a Ph.D. and not a medical degree. They are expert at administering tests of cognitive function, including memory, and interpreting the test results as normal or abnormal. They usually work in collaboration with a primary care physician, neurologist, or psychiatrist.

Where to Go for Help

Some doctors still advise their patients not to worry, that memory loss is just part of growing old and can't be helped. Clearly, they have not kept up with the latest developments that show how memory loss can be reversed or at least slowed down.

If you have severe memory loss then you should see a doctor. In our specialty center, neurologists, psychiatrists, and neuropsychologists work closely together, using a team approach. Until the average physician gets better at recognizing the types and causes of memory loss, your best option is to go to one of these specialized academic medical centers that employs a team approach. There are now a large number of these centers serving virtually every major urban, and even semiurban, area in the United States (listed in the appendix). If you do not have ready access to one of these centers, consult a neurologist or psychiatrist, or your primary care physician. Inquire if they have experience in diagnosing and treating memory loss and dementia.

If you have no memory loss, or mild memory loss not due to a specific reversible cause, you probably do not need to consult any physician and can go ahead with learning about and implementing the Memory Program in this book. But to identify exactly where you stand on the spectrum of memory loss, you need to take the following memory tests and see how well you perform on them.

Simple Tests to Check Your Memory

The questionnaire below is a modified version of a published scale (Gilewski et al., 1990) and is followed by two tests of memory. You should complete the questionnaire before attempting the memory tests.

Subjective Memory Questionnaire (Self-Administered)

This test requires five to ten minutes and should be completed by you without any help or interference from anyone else.

Globally, how would you rate your memory? In the row below, circle a number between 1 and 7 that best reflects your overall judgment about your memory.

No problem ⟵————————⟶ **Major problem**

1	2	3	4	5	6	7

The next two sets of questions have the same 1–7 scoring scheme for each item: 1=no problem, 2–3=mild problem, 4–5=moderate problem, 6–7=major problem.

General Frequency of Forgetting

In evaluating your own memory, how often do these present a problem for you? Circle a number between 1 and 7 for each item separately.

	No problem ⟵⟶ Major problem						
Remembering							
Names	1	2	3	4	5	6	7
Faces	1	2	3	4	5	6	7
Appointments	1	2	3	4	5	6	7
Where you put things, like keys	1	2	3	4	5	6	7
To perform household chores	1	2	3	4	5	6	7

Directions to places	1	2	3	4	5	6	7
Phone numbers just checked	1	2	3	4	5	6	7
Phone numbers frequently used	1	2	3	4	5	6	7
Things people tell you	1	2	3	4	5	6	7
To keep up correspondence	1	2	3	4	5	6	7
Personal dates (e.g., birthdays)	1	2	3	4	5	6	7
Words	1	2	3	4	5	6	7
What to buy in the store	1	2	3	4	5	6	7
How to take a test	1	2	3	4	5	6	7

Other Memory Problems

Starting a task, then forgetting it	1	2	3	4	5	6	7
Losing the thread of thought in conversation	1	2	3	4	5	6	7
Losing the thread of thought in public speaking	1	2	3	4	5	6	7
Not knowing if you've already told someone something	1	2	3	4	5	6	7

Use of Mnemonics

How often do you use these techniques to remind yourself about things?

	Rarely	←——→			Constantly		
Keep an appointment book	1	2	3	4	5	6	7
Write yourself reminder notes	1	2	3	4	5	6	7
Make lists of things to do	1	2	3	4	5	6	7
Make grocery lists	1	2	3	4	5	6	7

Plan your daily schedule in advance	1	2	3	4	5	6	7
Use mental repetition	1	2	3	4	5	6	7
Associate items with other things	1	2	3	4	5	6	7
Keep things you will need in a prominent place so as to notice them	1	2	3	4	5	6	7

Interpret Your Score

Now that you've completed this questionnaire, it's time to check the results. The first section, General Frequency of Forgetting, covers a number of areas that people commonly worry about with their memory. You can add up the total score and then divide by the number of items (eighteen in the first section) to get an average score on the 1 to 7 scale. If your average score is in the 1 to 2 range, your memory as measured by this scale is very good. If your average score is in the 5 to 7 range, then clearly these memory problems are interfering with your daily life.

If you have trouble remembering words or things that people tell you, you have poor verbal memory—information coded as words in the brain is not retained and retrieved well. In most people, verbal memory depends on proper functioning of the left half of the brain. If you scored 2 to 5 (or higher) for trouble remembering where you put your keys or losing your way when going to a place you've been before, your visuospatial or three-dimensional (3-D) memory is not up to the mark. In most people, this type of "nonverbal" memory depends on proper functioning of the right half of the brain.

The second part of the questionnaire evaluates the use of mnemonics and related techniques. Using mnemonics to compensate for a memory deficit may indicate a problem, but if you consciously use mnemonics to improve a basically sound memory, then scoring high on this part of the questionnaire doesn't mean very much. So the mnemonics section is harder to interpret than the first section.

There are other problems with all self-administered questionnaires of this type. Some worrywarts with an excellent memory will give themselves terrible scores, while others who blithely report no memory complaints on this questionnaire may score poorly on objective tests. So the self-administered memory questionnaire requires follow-up with objective memory tests in order to get a true picture.

Objective Memory Tests

Before you take these tests, you must recognize the difference between lack of attention and true memory loss. Poor attention leads to difficulty in registering the material presented in the test (or in real life), and if a fact isn't recorded in the brain it obviously cannot be recalled. This is quite different from true memory loss, where the material is registered and then recorded as a memory that resides in a group of nerve cells, but later the memory cannot be retrieved. So if you feel you cannot pay attention or concentrate because you are distracted, or have too many stresses in your life or worries on your mind, or suffer from depression, these tests can mislead you into believing that you have severe memory loss or dementia, when in fact the problem lies elsewhere. Therefore, *you must free yourself of all distractions and interference when you take these tests.*

The tests described here require a second person to administer them. Hints and prompts are not allowed during these tests, which is why it is sometimes better to ask someone other than a family member or close friend to be the tester. Ideally, the tests should be administered by trained neuropsychologists or other professionals, but they are simple enough for a nonprofessional to administer, as long as he or she carefully follows the required rules for administering the tests.

The tester should now take over and read the following sections, then administer the tests to you, one by one. Only after you've completed these tests are you allowed to read the remainder of this chapter. If you do not follow these instructions strictly, the tests are completely invalid. Therefore, if you're going to take these two tests, *ask the tester to carefully read the following section and understand what he/she needs to do before giving you the test. Stop reading here and hand this book over to the tester, who will need a pencil.*

Mini Mental State Examination

Tester: carefully read and understand the next two paragraphs, then give the test exactly as instructed in these two paragraphs.

The tester recites three unrelated objects (nouns)—for example, bus, door, rose (another option: apple, table, penny)—and the subject is required to repeat them back correctly.

Accuracy, not order, is what counts. The tester should circle the number of words correctly repeated by the subject at the first attempt.

Number of words repeated correctly (*first attempt only*)
0   1   2   3

Then the tester asks the subject to mentally subtract 7 serially from 100 (93, 86, 79, etc), and stop after five answers. After this test of calculation, which is meant to distract the subject from focusing on memorizing the three words, the tester tells the subject, "Repeat back the three words that I told you earlier." Again, absolutely no hints or prompts or extra conversation are permitted. Responses should be exact to get a positive score, and words that are similar in meaning (dime instead of penny) or spelling (tablet instead of table) should be given a score of 0. The tester should score only the subject's first attempt, based on how many of the original three words were accurately recalled.

Number of words recalled correctly (*first attempt only*)
0   1   2   3

End of Test

Tester: skip the next two paragraphs and proceed to List-Learning Test.

This is clearly a test of verbal memory. Recalling all three words accurately at the first attempt indicates that there are no major problems with your memory, while recalling 2 out of 3 words suggests that your memory may be a little shaky. Recalling only 1 word, or even worse, 0 out of 3 words, is not a good sign and should trigger clinical consultation. These recommendations flow partly from the results of a study that I published with my colleagues in 1997. In that study, seventy-five outpatients, who ranged in age from their forties to eighties, with minimal to mild cognitive impairment were followed for an average of two and a half years. People who recalled 0 or 1 out of 3 objects on this test were at high risk of developing dementia during follow-up, a score of 2 out of 3 was associated with low to moderate risk of developing dementia, and virtually no one who correctly scored 3 out of 3 met diagnostic criteria for dementia at the final follow-up visit. Other studies have also shown that this simple test is quite useful in distinguishing between people with mild versus severe memory disorders. The complete version of the Mini Mental State examination has a dozen items that covers a range of cognitive functions, with a maximum score of 30 (Folstein et al., 1975; see bibliography).

The next memory task is a little more difficult and is particularly useful in distinguishing normal memory from subtle memory loss.

Tester: read and understand this section (until "end of all tests") before actually giving the test.

List-Learning Test (brief version of standard tests)

The tester needs a pencil and paper, and access to a watch or clock.
     The tester gives the subject the following instruction: "I am going to read you a list of words. Listen carefully because when I'm through I want you to tell me all the words I read to you. The order in which you repeat the words does not matter. Are you ready?"
     The tester then reads the following list of words in a normal conversational voice at a steady pace, clearly pronouncing all the words.

cry	step	load
plate	pound	shirt
hip	blank	queen
fold	gift	teach

Immediately after reading this list, the tester says, "Now tell me every word in the list that you remember." As the subject recites the words, the tester checks them off against the list above. The tester scores the number of words correctly recalled. Near misses (for example, jacket instead of shirt or toad instead of load) are scored 0, and all other errors also get a 0. There is no minus scoring for wrong words (no penalty).

Number of words correctly recalled: _____
(range 0 to 12)

Then the subject is distracted (e.g., with conversation or by doing chores or other tasks) for the next fifteen minutes. Then the tester asks how many words the subject remembers from the original list of words. Using the same rules (near misses and wrong answers each get 0) as with the initial presentation, the number of words correctly recalled is noted.
     A key factor in this test is that the subject should not be given a warning that the list of words will need to be recalled fifteen minutes after the initial presentation.

End of All Tests

The subject is now allowed to resume reading this book.

You, the reader, should now go back and start reading again from the point where you stopped and handed the book over to the tester.

On the list of words test, the maximum score is 12. If you scored in the 8 to 12 range at the initial presentation (immediate recall) and recalled 6 to 12 words correctly fifteen minutes later (delayed recall), you have an excellent memory. Among people with average memory, those in their forties will usually recall 5 to 8 words after the fifteen-minute delay, while people in their sixties to seventies will usually get 4 to 6 words right on delayed recall. The delayed recall score is more important than the immediate recall score. Some people with a good memory don't pay enough attention to the initial list presentation but later are able to remember the majority of the words that they recited initially.

Interpreting Your Test Results

These memory tests are not foolproof and do not adequately substitute for neuropsychological testing, but they do provide a useful guide to categorize memory loss.

1. **NO MEMORY LOSS.** If you remembered 3 out of 3 objects on the MMS memory subtest and scored 5 or more on delayed recall on the 12-word list-learning task, you don't have memory loss. Nonetheless, as you grow older, there is a good chance that your memory will decline, even if it is sound right now. Therefore, I recommend that you read on and learn more about taking proactive action against future memory loss.
2. **SUBTLE TO MILD MEMORY LOSS.** If you recalled 2 out of 3 objects on the MMS, or if you had a delayed recall score of 3 to 4 on the list-learning task, you probably have subtle to mild memory loss. Note that scoring well on one (but not both) of the two tests still suggests subtle memory loss.
3. **SEVERE MEMORY LOSS.** If you remembered none or only 1 out of 3 objects on the MMS subtest, or had a delayed recall score of only 2 or less out of 12 words, you absolutely must go see your doctor, and the Memory Program is not for you. These recommendations also apply

to anyone else who takes these tests, for example, one of your parents.

Other Tests of Memory

The Selective Reminding Test is a complex list-learning test that starts in a simple way: the tester recites a list of twelve unrelated words and then asks the subject to recite all twelve words together. Then comes the tricky part: the tester prompts the subject with only those words that the subject missed on the first repetition, following which the subject is again required to repeat all twelve words, that is, recite the words that were missed the first time as well as those that were "kept in memory" from the first to the second trial. This sequence continues until the subject either gets all twelve words correct in successive repetitions or a total of twelve trials is completed. In the delayed recall part, the subject is challenged fifteen minutes after the last trial to recall the entire list of twelve words. The large number of trials requires complex scoring procedures and neuropsychological expertise. The Visual Reproduction subtest of the Wechsler Memory Scale is a different type of test because it evaluates the ability to remember shapes (recalling visual images).

Each test taps into a slightly different aspect of memory. A neuropsychologist typically administers a whole range of tests and looks for consistent patterns of deficits. If the subject performs well in all except one test, it may be due to a lapse in concentration. On the other hand, if someone scores consistently below normal on several memory tests, further investigation is necessary.

Factors That Affect Your Memory Test Performance

Three well-recognized factors can influence performance on memory tests: age, education, and gender.

Age

Since it is "normal" for memory test scores to worsen as people grow older, the standard test scores are adjusted downward to get the "norms" for that age group. Therefore, a "normal" ninety-year-old person may actually score worse on the standardized memory tests than a fifty-year-old person with moderate memory loss.

These age-adjusted test scores are used to help distinguish a clinical disorder from normal test performance within a particular age group. The flip side, of course, is the risk of dismissing worsening memory as "normal" for a person's age and doing nothing about it.

Education

People who are highly educated score much better on neuropsychological tests than people with low levels of education. You may recall that when my patient Frieda Kohlberg, who had a genius-level IQ, developed only very subtle memory deficits and otherwise tested at or above the normal range for someone her age, it was actually the first sign of Alzheimer's disease. But compared to other tests of intelligence and cognitive ability, memory is less affected by the subject's educational background.

Gender

You may be wondering about the third leg of the triad: age, education, and gender. In fact, there are subtle differences: women score slightly better on tests of verbal memory, and men score slightly better on tests of nonverbal memory (unusual shapes and diagrams that cannot be "coded" verbally for recall) and mathematical ability. However, these differences are very small and may result more from bias during the educational process than from a true genetic influence.

If You Get Neuropsychological Testing

If you get neuropsychological testing, you should find out from the neuropsychologist if the actual raw scores were used to make the interpretation or if they were adjusted for age and other factors. If you do well with or without age and education adjustments, your mental faculties are in excellent condition. If you need such adjustments to raise you into the normal range for people at your age and education level, then you probably have subtle age-related memory loss. If you score poorly, whether age and education adjustments are made, your memory loss is severe enough that you should go see a physician (if you haven't already).

Action Steps to Evaluate Your Memory

- Subjectively, is your memory worsening over time based on your own perception? Do others say that your memory is worsening?
- Use the lists in this chapter to check if you have symptoms of mild or severe memory loss, and if you have functional impairment due to memory loss.
- Identify your strengths and weaknesses, separating them into the verbal and nonverbal (spatial, 3-D) memory categories, based on the Subjective Memory Questionnaire.
- Have someone give you the memory tests in this chapter. Classify yourself according to the post-test instructions into one of three categories: no memory loss, subtle to mild memory loss, severe memory loss.
- If your memory has worsened considerably over time, or if you have symptoms of severe memory loss, or if you scored very poorly on the memory tests, you should consult a neurologist or psychiatrist, preferably with the input of a neuropsychologist. If you have access, go to the memory disorders clinic at your local major academic medical center.
- If your memory has not worsened considerably over time and you do not have severe symptoms and you scored well on the memory tests, or if you have only minimal to mild deficits on the memory tests, medical consultation is not essential. In essence, if you have no memory loss or mild memory loss, you should read further to understand and implement the Memory Program in your daily life.

Imaging Your Brain to Diagnose Memory Loss

While neuropsychological testing is critical to define the extent of memory loss, brain imaging is often more helpful in identifying the type of brain abnormality that may be causing the memory loss. Brain imaging techniques broadly fall into two categories: structural (CT and MRI) and functional (SPECT and positron-emission tomography, or PET).

Features of Scan	CT or CAT	MRI	SPECT	PET
What the scan evaluates	Structure of brain	Structure of brain	Blood flow	Glucose consumption
Time spent in scanner	20–30 minutes	25–40 minutes	30–45 minutes	45–60 minutes
Diagnostic use	Stroke, tumor, abscess	Stroke, tumor, abscess; possibly early Alzheimer's	Possibly early Alzheimer's	Possibly early Alzheimer's
Resolution (smallest identifiable brain region)	4–5 mm (one-fifth of an inch)	2–3 mm (one-tenth of an inch)	7–10 mm (one-third of an inch)	6–8 mm (one-fourth of an inch)
Radiation exposure	Moderate	None	Moderate	Moderate
Claustro-phobia (machine closely surrounds head)	Uncommon	Common	Uncommon	Sometimes
Intravenous injection	No	No	Yes	Yes
Availability	Widespread	Widespread	Common	Rare
Cost (approximate)	$200–500	$400–1,100	$400–800	$1,000–2,500

Structural brain imaging techniques are used to evaluate the structure, or anatomy, of the brain. Computerized axial tomography (CAT or CT) was the first such technique. Strangely enough, it was invented in the 1970s by researchers at EMI, a British music recording company that couldn't capitalize on it, although they did get the Nobel Prize for their invention. CT scanners take a large number of X rays in different planes and use computer technology to "reconstruct" the internal brain structure, which then becomes crystal clear to the viewer.

MRI works on a different principle. A strong magnetic field is applied around the head, and the distance traveled by individual protons (subatomic particles) in response to the magnetic field is measured in various parts of the brain. The MRI's computers use this information to produce clear, fine-grained images of internal brain structures. Unlike CT, MRI involves no radiation exposure. In any case, the risk of damage from radiation is low for the brain because it has few dividing or reproducing cells, making DNA damage unlikely.

Claustrophobia can develop in the MRI machine, which makes a loud banging noise. "Open" MRI is a method recently developed for people who have claustrophobia, but because it is open (the head is only partially enclosed) the magnetic field used is weaker and the sensitivity of the technique is much lower than that of a regular MRI.

Both SPECT and PET involve the intravenous injection of a radioactive tracer that is taken up by the brain. A combination of high-resolution cameras and sophisticated computers produces a 3-D image of radioactive tracer counts, representing blood flow or glucose metabolism (consumption), throughout the brain. SPECT or PET can reveal subtle deficits in blood flow or glucose consumption that have not led to changes in brain structure—the subject may still have a normal MRI. The first patient described in the introduction, David Finestone, had a subtle blood flow deficit on SPECT in the presence of a normal MRI, and this information proved very useful in his clinical management.

Brain Imaging to Diagnose Early Alzheimer's Disease

Recent studies show that a reduction in size of the hippocampus (which can be detected by using MRI) and a reduction in temporal and parietal lobe blood flow (SPECT) and glucose metabolism (PET) are often early diagnostic features of Alzheimer's disease. However, using MRI to assess the hippocampus requires sophisticated, labor-intensive research techniques (visual inspection isn't good enough). Also, these abnormalities detected by MRI and SPECT/PET can occur as part of normal aging and in other neurologic disorders. Although none of these techniques are diagnostic by themselves, they can help when the clinical picture is unclear.

Functional MRI is a new technique that involves looking at changes in hemoglobin oxygen saturation (indicates brain tissue oxygen use), usually while the subject is performing a test of attention or memory. Functional MRI is in its infancy but may well become the wave of the future. A major problem is that its results are worthless if people cannot keep their heads completely still while they lie in the scanner.

The decision about which brain imaging technique to use remains in the hands of your physician. Nonetheless, if you have memory loss, knowing the basics outlined here will make you a more informed consumer about the role of these brain imaging procedures in diagnosing the cause of your memory loss.

CHAPTER 2

How Your Brain Remembers— and Forgets

Memory storage in the brain is not like a videotape that we can wind or unwind at will. New learning, old information, and the links between them are constantly formed and destroyed in a dynamic process.

Implicit versus Explicit Memory

Memory can be classified into implicit and explicit categories. When you open your car door, turn on the ignition, and start driving, do you actually make a conscious effort to remember how to perform this sequence of actions? Of course not. The memory of how to drive a car is already hardwired and automatic, and you usually don't need to pay any attention to it. The memory of how to drive a car required conscious "explicit" mental effort when you first took driving lessons, but it is now "implicit" or automatic. This "macro" memory with many hardwired components has room for flexibility—for example, when you drive a rental car or a friend's automobile. It takes you a couple of moments to adjust to the new vehicle, to identify the positioning of the dashboard and driving controls, but soon you get the hang of it and you're off without a care in the world. But your macro memory of how to drive a car cannot make huge shifts, as any automobile driver who tries to ride a motorbike for the first time can testify. So the nerve cells that store this information are not made of concrete or steel, but neither are they like a bowl of jelly—maybe more like a hard lump of Plasticine that changes its shape only with considerable force.

Skills and habits come under implicit memory. Classical conditioning and other types of memory, which also fall into this implicit category, are related to simple reflex reactions, for example, jumping away when touching a hot object, that we execute automatically in our everyday lives. But when you think of "memory," you probably think of something else altogether: discrete events, like recalling someone's birthday or where you went on vacation a few years ago. This type of memory is called "episodic" or "event-related" or "explicit" memory. You have to make a conscious effort to retrieve the explicit memory of a fact or event, unlike the implicit memory of knowing how to drive a car. In this book, I generally use the word *memory* as it is commonly understood: explicit memory of both short-term and long-term specific events.

For explicit memory, there are three elements to the sequence of remembering:

1. Acquiring information. Attention and concentration are key.
2. Storing the event or episode as a memory. Importance, meaning, and emotional impact of the event determine if the brain will store it as a memory.
3. Retrieval. This is the active process of bringing the memory into the forefront of consciousness.

Facts about the Human Brain
- It makes up 2 percent of body weight.
- It consumes 25 percent of the body's glucose and oxygen for its energy needs.
- It contains around 100 billion neurons, also called nerve cells.
- Each neuron communicates via chemical messengers with hundreds of other nerve cells.
- The brain may contain up to 60 trillion pieces of memory.
- Mainly short-term, and some long-term, memories are located in the hippocampus and other parts of the temporal lobe.
- Many long-term memories have migrated from the hippocampus to reside in the frontal lobe.
- Loss of nerve cells in the temporal lobe, and in parts of the frontal lobe, leads to memory loss.

Short-Term versus Long-Term Memory

Explicit memory can be short-term (seconds to hours) or long-term (days to years). Short-term memory has limited capacity, but long-term memory has a lot of available disk space to store data. A simple example illustrates this point: you may find it difficult to repeat more than two new telephone numbers recited consecutively to you, but you can easily recall several telephone numbers that are in long-term storage in your brain. This simple fact tells you that the mechanisms by which the brain stores short-term and long-term memories must be different.

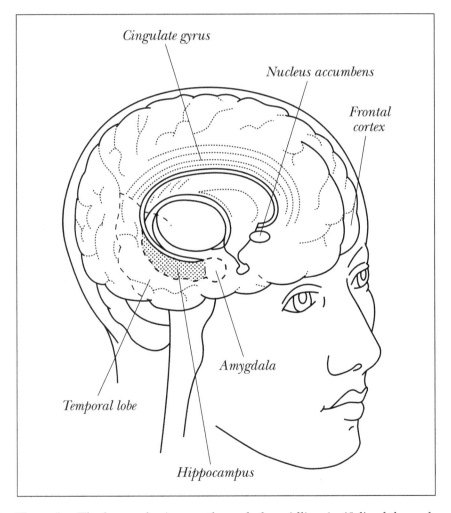

Figure 1. The human brain seen through the midline (as if sliced through the middle of the face to the middle of the back of the head).

Hippocampus: Grand Central Station of Memory

The hippocampus is a wing-shaped, inch-long structure that makes up the inner part of the temporal lobe. The temporal lobe is a bigger structure, the size of a large kiwi fruit or oblong plum, that projects from the lower front part of the brain and lies just beneath the side, or temple, of the forehead. The brain is divided into two big halves, so the right hippocampus is part of the right temporal lobe, and the left hippocampus is part of the left temporal lobe.

Nerve impulses from our senses first pass through a filter that screens the information and ignores what is unimportant. If the information survives this first gauntlet, it is sent via nerve cells to the hippocampus and surrounding regions. Each specialized neuron in the hippocampus records an element of the fact or event, and these nerve cells link all the components together to form a composite memory trace. This memory trace is housed in thousands of nerve cells, probably in proteins and ribonucleic acids (RNA).

How Short-Term Converts to Long-Term Memory

If the memory is important enough, or if the same event repeats many times over a long period, the short-term memory trace residing within these hippocampal nerve cells is eventually moved into permanent, long-term storage. The hippocampus has broad-band connections— fiber optic rather than regular copper wire—to the frontal lobes, where many long-term memories are stored (some long-term memories remain in the hippocampus).

The Web of Memory

Each memory is a complex web of material that mixes facts, sensations, and emotions. When a strong emotion accompanies an event, you release more of the chemical transmitters that communicate among nerve cells to help form memories. Emotional states represent an important "internal" environmental cue for memory. Think of the emotion-laden memories that flooded through your mind at your graduation, your wedding, when you had major conflicts with family members, or when you lost someone close to you. These memories stay hardwired forever in your brain, ready to be recalled whenever the occasion arises. On the other hand, you remember only fragments of less important and less emotional events, such as the details of a boring business trip or meeting; the threads of the spider's web have broken because of lack of interest and disuse.

Over time, long-term memory tends to get pushed from consciousness into the subconscious. Then a simple cue, an odd association, a chance meeting, can activate the sleeping spider's web and fire the neuronal circuits, resurrecting the long-term memory that had seemingly evaporated from your mind.

Your Brain Is Plastic

If your skin is cut superficially, it heals within a few days. Many other organs in the body can also repair themselves: new cells are generated by cells that divide and reproduce in response to injury. Unfortunately, while brain cells do grow and specialize during infancy and childhood, by the time we become adults nearly all of them lose the capacity to divide and reproduce. And yet we know that our brains are constantly changing: we learn throughout our lives, we have a range of reactions that we can modulate in response to other people, places, and even time itself. So how do we explain this contradiction: the brain creates no new nerve cells but has great flexibility? The answer lies in the revolutionary new finding of brain plasticity.

Dr. Eric Kandel, a Nobel Prize winner, works a few floors above my office in the same research institute. For several decades, Kandel has studied a species of snail called *aplysia,* which looks like a small black blob with ears. *Aplysia* has large nerve cells that lend themselves to experiments. Kandel's groundbreaking studies have shown that many nerve cells in *aplysia,* and in more complex species, retain the property of plasticity, which means that they can change their structure or function over time. The nerve cells do this by sprouting new branches called dendrites and forming contacts with other nerve cells to compensate for those that have been lost. Using a different approach, Bruce McEwen's laboratory at Rockefeller University demonstrated what was once thought to be impossible: plasticity and regeneration of nerve cells in the hippocampus in animal studies.

As an analogy, we know that people who are born blind develop an exquisite sense of touch and hearing. For those who constantly use Braille and become expert at it, the brain region responsible for controlling the one finger used for reading physically grows in size. This type of compensation may also occur following memory loss, depending on the cause.

Are There Limits to Your Memory?

Is there a limit to how much you can remember? Off hand, we all know that we *can* teach an old dog new tricks. Millions of people who are past their so-called prime are able to take college courses and graduate with advanced degrees. But if there are distinct brain regions for each subtype of memory—proper nouns versus other nouns, for example—don't these bookshelves get saturated over a lifetime of exposure to thousands of pieces of information that make up our brain libraries? And if these brain regions get saturated, how can a middle-aged or older person still have the capacity to learn whole new languages and technologies?

The answer is simple: memory is a dynamic, not a static, process. There are several ways by which your memory storage keeps expanding:

1. As you learn more, and learn more efficiently, the nerve cells responsible for memory develop new tricks and become more expert at importing new knowledge into the available nerve cells.
2. Few of us have taxed our memories to such an extent that all the memory nerve cells are clogged up and overflowing with knowledge, though if you're a quiz or game show expert you may come fairly close.
3. Finally, there is an obvious solution when you need more memory: drag the useless stuff to the trash, choose "empty trash" from the pop-up menu, and a few megabytes of memory storage immediately open up in your brain.

CHAPTER 3

How Aging Affects
Your Memory

If a young or middle-aged man, when leaving
company, does not recollect where he laid his hat, it is
nothing; but if the same inattention is discovered in an
old man, people will shrug up their shoulders and say,
"His memory is going."
—SAMUEL JOHNSON

AGE-RELATED MEMORY LOSS occurs in all mammals, from mice to
humans. Research has narrowed down the myriad biological theories
of aging into a few that are backed by scientific evidence: genetically
programmed cell death, disruption of biological clocks, and free radical toxicity.

Programmed Death of Cells

The theory of programmed cell death states that every cell in the
body is genetically programmed to die at a certain point in time, and
that this time frame is specific for each type of cell. Many cells in the
body regularly die, but other reproducing cells make up the deficit.
Erythrocytes, or red blood cells, that carry hemoglobin have an average life span of only 120 days, but stem cells in the bone marrow continually develop into new erythrocytes and enter the bloodstream to

make up for this loss. But in cells that do not reproduce and are meant to last a lifetime, especially those in the brain, programmed cell death may play a major role. Just as there are genes that tell each cell to synthesize the right kinds of proteins to maintain life, other genes are programmed to turn off protein synthesis and destroy the cell. Currently, we do not know what triggers these "suicide" genes to come alive as we grow older. If the genes that trigger programmed cell death are successfully blocked, the human life span can be greatly prolonged. But what will society be like if new genetic therapies make people live to the age of 150 or 200 years? If in addition to increased longevity there is a corresponding improvement in quality of life, then the ensuing problems won't be as overwhelming as we now imagine.

Biological Clocks

Programmed cell death is like the entire assembly line going on permanent strike, leading to factory closure. Disruption of biological clocks is the entire managerial staff, including the chairman and board of directors, calling it quits. Many of the natural ebbs and flows in the body—including sleep, body temperature, and hormone secretion—are under the control of biological clocks that are genetically programmed to react according to set time sequences, such as the twenty-four-hour day, based on environmental inputs. As our DNA decays with aging, these natural rhythms become erratic and begin to desynchronize, weakening our natural defenses against disease. Gradually, over time, the disruption of biological clocks becomes a central feature of the aging process.

By itself, this theory does not explain why we age the way we do. Many bodily functions do not have natural biological clocks, and only a few of the brain's functions, particularly sleep, are under this type of rhythmic control. Even the heart, a structure that requires near-perfect rhythmic performance to ensure survival, is not affected very much by circadian (twenty-four-hour) rhythms.

Free Radicals Are Toxic

That's what some people said in the 1960s and 1970s. But jokes aside, what exactly are free radicals? Free radicals are formed when an atom or molecule carries an unpaired electron. This extra negative electrical charge launches a cascade of chemical reactions that eventually lead to cell death. Free radicals are constantly produced by chemical reactions throughout the body, and both stress and a diet high in saturated fats increase free radical formation. The most common free radicals are hydrogen peroxide, which is formed when a molecule of water gets an extra oxygen atom, as well as oxygen itself.

Oxygen is essential for life, but the addition of an unpaired electron makes it toxic to cells in the body. Dr. Jekyll turns into Mr. Hyde, and life-giving oxygen metamorphoses into a merciless killer.

If toxic free radicals are continually being formed in our bodies, how do we survive? As with everything else, nature has provided a counterbalance to deal with this threat. Enzymes called free radical scavengers, notably superoxide dismutase, routinely destroy the free radicals that are formed. These enzymes decline with age, and a gradual imbalance develops, with free radicals gaining the upper hand. Many therapies are based on the idea that decreasing free radical toxicity will slow down the aging process. For example, vitamin E is the most widely used antioxidant, and it destroys the bad oxygen when it appears in the body. Melatonin also possesses some antioxidant properties, as does the prescription medication selegiline (Deprenyl). These substances can help prevent the ravages of the aging process, and memory loss in particular.

Genes versus Environment

Some people have an excellent memory for words, others for numbers, and still others for music. But are there genes that regulate how the brain ages? Do genes give us our memory power during our youth? And as we age, to what extent do genes control or program the time when nerve cells degenerate in the hippocampus and frontal lobes? We are waiting for the answers to these questions, because only then will it become possible to translate this genetic knowledge into practical, therapeutic interventions.

George Burns drank like a fish, smoked like a chimney, and did a few more exciting things on the side. Nevertheless, he lived to be over a hundred; obviously he had good longevity genes. Inherent genetic variability influences not only longevity but also intellectual functions and memory, so that a fifty-year-old may have the brain of an eighty-five-year-old, and vice versa. But in addition to genetic influences, environmental factors can magnify, and sometimes directly cause, memory loss as you grow older. These effects can be directly altered, unlike your genes. I will focus on these environmental, usually reversible, factors in a later section in this book.

Aging Weakens Recent Memory

Do you remember what you ate for lunch today? How about yesterday? And how about a week ago? For most of you, whatever happened today is still in active memory, yesterday is hovering above the "memory trash," and the meal from a week ago is already in the trash and likely gone for good. The time factor is crucial; as you go further back in time, memories begin to vanish. The paradox is that as you grow older, it is not the old memories that disappear but more often the recent ones. Most recent memories—even if they are closer to consciousness and hence more "active"—are not hardwired in your brain as firmly as old memories, so you can understand why lapses in recent memory occur during the aging process.

The Power of Learning

When infant mice are made to learn a complex task like traversing a maze to reach a source of food, the process leads to increased branching and connectivity among nerve cells in the brain. Learning literally leads to a structural change in nerve cells in the mouse brain, and these changes can become permanent, resulting in superior memory and intelligence. In children, we call this education. In the mice experiments, the branching of dendrites slows down and then stops as age advances, so that new learning becomes more limited. Similarly, in people, the ability to learn new information is greatest during childhood and decreases in later life when nerve cells lose their capacity to grow and branch out to form new contacts with other nerve cells. This topic reminds me of an incident that taught me a great deal about our capacity to learn, and how this changes as we grow older.

Back when I was at Yale, I met Anil Deolalikar, an economist who was then a junior faculty member. Later, he got married and settled down in Seattle. When I visited him there, his daughter was barely three years old. One morning, he played a game in which he showed her several large cards filled with red polka dots closely packed across the white surface. One card had sixty-seven dots, another sixty-nine, a third seventy-one, and so on. Each time he flashed the card in front of her, she would immediately blurt out the right number of dots. For the life of me, I couldn't make out the differences between the number of red dots on these cards, and neither could Anil. I was impressed, because clearly his three-year-old daughter wasn't familiar with the concept of numbers, let alone the meaning of sixty-nine or seventy-one. Anil explained to me that his daughter wasn't really unique—very young children normally possess a nearly perfect visual photographic memory. This ability is lost when they grow older, perhaps because it is displaced by the development of language.

This experience increased my awareness of the fact that there are many untapped resources within each one of us. Cultivating these skills is essential to developing and maintaining our intellectual faculties, including memory. Even though prime time for learning is when you are young, learning and memory can still be enhanced in middle age and beyond, provided you undertake the right steps.

What Is Senility?: Esther's Story

Esther Erickson, an eighty-three-year-old retired bookkeeper living alone, came with a long-standing friend and neighbor who had persuaded Esther that her memory needed to be checked. Esther had begun to forget names, locked herself out of her apartment a couple of times, and had accidentally left the stove on once. Other than a slight slowness in walking, there wasn't anything unusual in her neurological examination, and her psychiatric assessment was completely normal. The rest of my diagnostic workup was notable for only two findings. Her memory was slightly below par, but otherwise she scored in the normal range for someone her age on the neuropsychological tests. Her MRI scan revealed a very small stroke in the basal ganglia, which is a brain center that controls motor movements. This helped explain her slowness in walking but not her memory lapses.

Before I complete her story, put on your diagnostic hat for a moment. Is this normal aging? Is this mild memory loss? Or is this early Alzheimer's disease? And where does "senility" fit into the picture?

Esther Erickson does not fit well into any diagnostic category. She is precisely the kind of patient who would have been rated as being on the way to "senility" if she had come to see a doctor fifty years ago. Nowadays, we don't like to use the term senility because it blurs the distinctions between mild memory loss and dementia. Also, the old concept of senility implied that it was caused by hardening or blocking of arteries and their smaller branches. However, recent research has shown that age-related memory loss is usually not caused by diseases of arteries or other blood vessels in the brain.

A year later, Esther died suddenly of a heart attack. The brain autopsy showed no evidence of stroke other than in the basal ganglia, consistent with the clinical and MRI results. The only other abnormality was an occasional amyloid plaque without any neurofibrillary tangles. Amyloid plaques and neurofibrillary tangles, both of which are visible only under a microscope, are the pathologic features of Alzheimer's disease. But with aging, an occasional amyloid plaque can appear even in the absence of any symptoms of memory loss. So while her autopsy told us that she did not have Alzheimer's disease, we couldn't rule out the possibility that it would have developed if she had lived for another five to ten years.

I think it is best to drop the term senility because it doesn't tell us anything beyond the fact that the person is old and has memory loss.

What Aging Is and Isn't

Dr. Robert Butler, formerly the head of the department of geriatric medicine at Mount Sinai School of Medicine in New York, cautioned against "ageism," which is a tendency to think of every problem of the elderly as being a natural consequence of aging and hence doing nothing to solve it. Ageism also underlies the widespread prejudice against older people and is sometimes used to prevent them from working, or forcing them to retire early.

Aging does not mean you have to:

- Lose interest in doing things.
- Lose your memories permanently.
- Get depressed.
- Focus on death more than on life.
- Think that it is no longer possible to change.
- Be satisfied with being bored.
- View the rest of your life as a downhill course.

Successful aging involves:

- A positive outlook.
- Continuing to maintain interests and hobbies.

- Looking forward to change and having a willingness to adapt.
- Maintaining strong relationships and social bonds.
- Maintaining high self-esteem.
- Bouncing back from adversity.

Young Learning, Old Learning

Aging has a gradual, steadily progressive impact on memory processes. Compared to young people, older people are less skilled in associating unrelated items presented to them. This decline is greatest when older subjects have to associate different stimuli to produce a complex memory, and is probably due to loss of nerve cells in the association areas (brain regions responsible for associating different events and stimuli) in the parahippocampus and the frontal lobes. However, in these same experiments, older people were much better than their young counterparts at tasks requiring planning, organization, and the manipulation of information. In other words, even though young adults are much better at learning new information than middle-aged and older people, they fall short when it comes to tasks that require careful planning and judgment. You should recognize this organizational capacity as an important strength in yourself when you evaluate your intellectual capabilities.

Aging Changes Your Mental Abilities
- Reaction time to an event slows
- Dealing with multiple stimuli and tasks becomes difficult
- Thinking slows
- Learning new information becomes difficult
- Remembering names becomes more difficult
- Short-term memory slowly deteriorates
- Intelligence and long-term memory are preserved, including memory for music and other artistic memories
- Common sense, planning, organizational skills, and judgment improve. You develop wisdom.

Creativity and Associative Thinking

The flip side of cognitive decline is cognitive improvement, and further along the spectrum lies the phenomenon of creativity. Some creative abilities are innate or genetic, like musical skills, but learning and practice are necessary to develop such talents. Associative thinking, which is controlled by the parahippocampus and parts of the frontal lobe, involves taking a new piece of information and linking it to another piece of data that lies stored in memory. We all do this from time to time, but the creative person tends to do it more often and can sometimes take big leaps by connecting ideas that many would consider to be quite distinct and separate. The creative individual recognizes the importance of this new connection, builds on it, and is off and running.

Einstein's Brain

Therefore, from a theoretical perspective, the association areas in the parahippocampus and the frontal lobes should be better developed in highly creative people. The initial autopsy evaluation of Albert Einstein's brain revealed that it was a normal size, and the association areas in his cerebral cortex were not large. But a recent reexamination showed that his brain lacked the Sylvian fissure, which borders the temporal lobe, and had a slight enlargement in the lower part of the temporal lobe near the association areas. These results were given big play in the media, but they don't really resolve any issues. Maybe Einstein wasn't the best prototype to study, because he made quantum leaps to develop entirely new fields virtually from scratch, leaving bread-and-butter associative thinkers behind in the dust. Maybe the unique connections within his brain were simply beyond the detection capability of standard neuropathologic methods.

The Nobel Prize: Old Winners, Young Winners

In general, aging does have a negative impact on creativity, and this is probably due to the decay in association cortex nerve cells over time. Nobel Prize winners invariably complete their groundbreaking work in their thirties and forties, although the rest of the world may take a few decades to catch on and give them their just reward. But creativity does not disappear as you grow older. Rather, it gets modified by a lifetime of experience that results in your balancing new ideas with common sense and judgment, leading to what is commonly called wisdom. As a matter of fact, some people continue to be creative even after developing severe memory loss. After Willem de

Kooning developed Alzheimer's disease, he remained a productive painter into his eighties and nineties. The quality of his paintings changed, and the precise line of his brush strokes became blurry. The art critics, who were unaware of his brain disorder, announced a new creative phase in the painter's career.

PART TWO

Start the Memory Program

CHAPTER 4

Put Together Your Memory Program

Principles of the Memory Program

1. You need to adopt a comprehensive memory program rather than hope for a quick fix against age-related memory loss.
2. No single approach will be sufficient to prevent memory loss due to aging, or to block or reverse age-related memory loss after it has set in. An integrated approach that includes sound general health measures (diet, exercise, memory training), identifying and reversing specific causes of memory loss for those who have such causes, and limited use of medications (vitamins, alternative therapies, and pharmaceuticals) will give you the maximum benefit.
3. The program requires consistency and long-term commitment, because given the nature of age-related memory loss, you may not see any results for many months or even years after you begin the program.
4. You don't need to follow every single suggestion or piece of advice; rather, you should tailor the program to your own needs. For example, while everyone should develop sound dietary and exercise habits, not everyone needs to take medications to prevent memory loss. The Memory Program itself is individualized and tailor-made for people in specific age

and gender categories, with separate guidelines for those who wish to prevent memory loss versus those who already have mild memory loss and need to treat it and prevent further decline.

In this chapter, I introduce the basic outline of the Memory Program. In subsequent chapters, I go through the various elements that constitute the Memory Program, giving you a detailed description and explanation of the science and clinical basis behind the practical recommendations, and how you should go about making the decision to implement each component in your own life. I then bring all this information together in a chapter devoted to describing the Memory Program in detail. I urge you to read this book sequentially and not skip to the later chapter that describes the program itself, because much of what you need there won't be clear if you haven't read the earlier chapters.

If You're Not Sure

If your memory is sound and you have excellent general health habits, you might justifiably ask why you need to even bother about age-related memory loss. My answer is quite simple: if you are willing to suffer a gradual dwindling in your memory starting in your forties and fifties, and continuing into your sixties and seventies, then you should not waste any of your time or energy worrying about it. But you probably belong to the majority of people who look forward to their golden years with hope and a positive attitude. You want to function at your peak physical and mental capacity for the longest possible period of time, so that your later years will truly be golden. If you belong to this group, now is the right time to begin taking steps to prevent age-related memory loss.

Don't Wait Until It Is Too Late

Prevention is the best strategy against the aging process, but our society often prefers to ignore problems until they strike us in the face. In some cases, we can get away with it, as the United States government managed to do with the federal budget deficit in the 1990s, waiting for the other shoe to drop before swinging into a corrective action mode. But maintaining good health is a different matter altogether.

Taking preventive action in your forties and fifties is a whole lot better than waking up for the first time in your sixties or seventies to discover that you've developed memory loss, a condition that gradually crept up on you while you ignored it. After age-related memory loss has set in, taking action at a late stage is not very effective because the death of nerve cells in the brain is largely irreversible. All that can be done is to prevent further damage, not rescue what has already been lost.

The Lessons of Osteoporosis and High Blood Pressure

The majority of older people, especially most women, gradually develop osteoporosis, which is a thinning and weakening of bone structure. If everyone said that there was no point in trying to prevent osteoporosis by using medications (estrogen, calcitonin, Fosamax, Evista) because it was, after all, "normal aging," you can imagine how frail and stooped most elderly women would be and how many more falls and fractures would occur. Hypertension is another such example: a mild to moderate rise in blood pressure was usually left untreated on the grounds that it was quite "normal" for an older person. After doctors began to treat even mild hypertension routinely, using diet, exercise, and medications if necessary (this practice began barely two to three decades ago), the risk of heart disease, stroke, and death in these people diminished steadily over time. Mild hypertension is now considered a treatable, and not just normal, part of the aging process. The same holds true for high cholesterol levels. The next sea change: preventing memory loss due to the aging process.

Grandma Still Has a Great Memory

But what evidence is there to support the dim view that most people will suffer from memory loss as they grow older? As a matter of fact, there has been considerable research on this topic. While a few people retain a stellar memory into their eighties and nineties, studies of middle-aged and older people consistently demonstrate that the vast majority show a gradual decline in their memory over time. When someone says that his or her grandmother has an outstanding memory, it usually means that her memory is much better than that of other people of her age, but it may still represent a decline from when she was younger. This is what we have observed in the Memory Disorders Center at Columbia University. Therefore, since age-related memory loss is likely to affect most of you in the years to come, you should begin to implement preventive strategies at this stage. And if you already have mild memory loss, you should get started on the Memory Program immediately.

The Three Main Elements in the Memory Program

There are three broad components to the Memory Program that I will describe in detail in the rest of this book:

1. Proactive general health measures that include a proper diet with appropriate nutritional supplements, regular moderate physical exercise, and practical training aids and techniques to boost your ability to remember.
2. Identifying specific causes of memory loss, many of which can be completely reversed if treated correctly. These include depression, stress, alcohol, hormonal abnormalities, nutritional deficiencies, and brain toxicity resulting from specific over-the-counter and prescription medications. Preventing stroke, particularly ministrokes, is another important element in this part of the Memory Program.
3. Medications to improve your memory. These include a variety of promemory medications—alternative, over-the-counter, and prescription. Some of them are useful in preventing or treating mild memory loss, others have questionable utility, and still others either don't work or are too toxic to use on a daily basis. I will review the evidence for and against each of these medications to help provide a sound basis for their inclusion or exclusion from the Memory Program.

Reversible and Less Reversible Memory Loss

All three sections of the Memory Program are important. Most of you will accept the idea that a sound diet with moderate, regular physical exercise supplemented by memory training techniques will help protect against memory loss. Some of you may also recognize the value of taking medications of one sort or another. But those who have a specific, reversible cause of memory loss are of particular concern to me. Depression is an obvious example, because it is often unrecognized by both the person suffering from this problem and the physician. Another common, often unidentified, culprit is alcohol, because with age the brain becomes more sensitive to even small doses—for example, your regular two to three drinks every evening can gradually cause brain toxicity as you grow older. Therefore, although only a minority among you will have a reversible cause of memory loss, if you do belong to this category it is imperative that the specific cause be identified and tackled head-on. And if you suffer from memory loss due to a reversible cause, general health improvement or memory training techniques or memory-enhancing medications won't do you much good until the actual cause is treated appropriately—for example, no amount of diet or exercise or memory training or promemory medications will cure memory loss if it is caused by thyroid deficiency; thyroid hormone replacement therapy is required.

I am emphasizing potentially reversible causes of memory loss precisely because they can often be fully reversed. For the more common problem of age-related memory loss, neither general health measures nor specific medications provide a perfect solution. These approaches will help slow down or block further decline in your memory, but they are unlikely to bring your memory back to what it was when you were twenty years old. This key fact makes it all the more important that you consider adopting this Memory Program before you develop significant memory loss.

If You Already Have Mild Memory Loss

Some of you have already developed mild age-related memory loss, based on either your performance in the memory tests that I described in the first chapter, or your own awareness that your memory is significantly worse compared to how it used to be a few years ago. But even if you fall into the category of those with mild memory loss, you can still employ components of the Memory Program with good results. Although people in their forties and fifties will benefit the most by adopting all the elements in the Memory Program, those among you who are sixty-plus will also gain by using these approaches.

Customize Your Memory Program

You should tailor the Memory Program to your own needs. For example, it is too expensive and cumbersome, and doesn't make a whole lot of sense, to take a medication cocktail of ginkgo biloba, vitamins A, C, and E, donepezil (Aricept), phosphatidylserine, selegiline, a COX II inhibitor like Celebrex or Vioxx, melatonin, and estrogen. Rational, practical choices among these various options are required. I will discuss the pros and cons of these choices, taking into account differences among individuals that will include a careful analysis of the risk-benefit ratio for each one of you. In the chapter that describes the entire Memory Program in detail later in the book, the optimal strategies within the program are specifically targeted for different groups of people:

1. People with mild memory loss versus people with currently normal memory who wish to prevent future loss.
2. People in the age group forty to fifty-nine versus those who are sixty and older, each described separately for the above two groups.
3. Men and women, described separately for each of the above categories.

This classification will help you develop and implement an individualized program for yourself to fight age-related memory loss. Before you go through the rest of the book, you should be clear as to whether you have a normal memory or already suffer from mild memory loss. Base this judgment mainly on your memory test performance in chapter 1 and don't rely only on your own subjective evaluation or the opinions of family and friends. I frequently return to this distinction in the rest of the book, and knowing whether you have a normal memory or mild memory loss will help you decide which advice does and does not apply to you.

CHAPTER 5

Start a Healthy Promemory Diet and Exercise Plan

A Case of Mayonnaise

When I joined Columbia University in 1985, I worked with a nurse who was, to put it mildly, overweight. One afternoon, I stopped by her desk to ask her a question and found her preparing for a well-deserved lunch. First, she brought out an enormous bowl of salad, full of greens, a few carrots thrown in for color. The gargantuan portion didn't faze me, because I had already been in the United States for five years and had become quite familiar with American eating habits. Actually, I was pleasantly surprised by her rigor in selecting such a healthy salad with essentially no fat in it. For a moment, I began to wonder why she was so bulky when her diet was so exemplary. But not for long. From another plastic bowl that she had brought from home, she unleashed several heaping spoonfuls of a thick, yellow-white salad dressing that looked like pure mayonnaise. I casually chatted with her about a patient we were treating, but I couldn't keep my eyes off the salad bowl. Rest assured, I had no interest whatsoever in sharing her meal; rather, it was the incongruity between the overgrown, leafy salad and the heavy, viscous dressing that struck me.

For years, I have watched such odd maneuvers with the distant curiosity of a physician who includes dietary advice as a prime component in his repertoire. But a few years ago, one of these newfangled culinary approaches struck a raw nerve in me.

Aggressive Dieting May Carry Risks: Lou's Story

A fifty-two-year-old psychiatrist-friend of mine, Lou, has always had a weight problem. So when I visited him and his family in suburban Westchester County, New York, in early 1998, I was quite surprised by what I saw. He had lost at least thirty pounds, and while not yet slim, he was getting pretty close. Lou proudly informed me that he was on a protein-rich and fatty food diet with no carbohydrates. No cereal, wheat, corn, rice, pasta, sugar, or potatoes. It seemed like an unnatural challenge to the normal course of healthy bodily metabolism, but I was pleased by his successful effort to shed a few pounds. In fact, more than a few.

A month later, I got a frantic telephone call from his wife, who informed me that her husband had just suffered a full-blown heart attack. I dropped what I was doing to help her during this emergency. Her husband underwent a balloon angioplasty and was able to gradually get back to work within a few weeks. "Low-carb" is now a taboo word in conversations in their house, because she feels that the diet precipitated her husband's heart attack. My friend also happens to have a strong family history of heart disease, making it hard to determine exactly what caused his heart attack. Given this uncertainty, I cannot say that the diet was the culprit. However, from a physiologic standpoint, we know that most cells in the body, and nearly all the cells in the brain, use carbohydrates like glucose or other simple sugars like fructose and galactose as their main energy source. For fats and proteins to be used as an energy source, they first have to be converted to glucose by specialized enzymes that parade up and down a series of dancing biochemical pathways. A diet that excludes carbohydrates puts extra pressure on the enzymes that lubricate this chemical maze, and they are now forced to work overtime on fats and proteins instead of on the carbohydrates that they prefer to face. This upsetting of the normal balance leads to weight loss, which can be dramatic, as occurred in my friend's case.

A Memory-Healthy Diet

Contrast these drastic tactics to the methods used by David Finestone, the forty-nine-year-old corporate executive that I described in the introduction. He came to see me with the symptom of forgetting names and appeared to have suffered from a very small stroke. Based on my advice, he lost weight by cutting back on his intake of saturated fats, primarily red meat and pizza. His program also included eating more fresh fruit and green vegetables, in addition to beginning regular physical exercise. Over time, these changes worked wonders for him. A sensible diet supplemented by a regular exercise regimen is by far the best strategy to lose weight. Why this simple, conventional approach is shunned by so many has always mystified me; perhaps they want a quick fix rather than wait for the slower, but more permanent, results from a long-term program.

Avoid Saturated Fats

A saturated fat–rich diet can indirectly lead to memory loss. High cholesterol levels lead to fatty plaques that deposit themselves on the inner walls of arteries and slow down blood flow in the brain. If this slowing of flow occurs in a small artery (as is common), blood clots gradually form and cause a ministroke, and depending on which part of the brain is damaged, cognitive deficits can occur. If hippocampal or specific frontal lobe nerve cells are affected, memory loss will be the result. The best time to focus on dietary preventive techniques is before these lesions develop, because after a ministroke, the dead nerve cells cannot be regenerated. Another reason for cutting back on saturated fats is that they increase the number of free radicals, which are toxic to most brain cells and can produce memory loss.

What's Good for Your Heart Is Good for Your Brain

A diet that is good for the heart is equally good for the brain. Foods that are low in saturated fats and high in fiber content and vitamins and minerals are ideal to prevent heart disease and stroke, and decrease free radical formation. The following table provides a broad overview of common foods and their relative nutritional content, and their potential impact on memory. Butter, margarine, and desserts are among the worst offenders, as is red meat. I strongly advise you to cook with oils high in unsaturated fats: canola, sunflower, corn, or olive oil. Walnuts contain a lot of "good" cholesterol and unsaturated

Common Foods and Their Nutritional Content

Foods	Fat Content	Protein Content	Carbohydrate Content	Vitamins	Minerals	Potential Impact on Memory
Butter, margarine	High	Nil	Nil	Nil	Nil	– –
Desserts	High	High	Medium to high	Low	Low	– –
Red meat (pork, beef)	High	High	Low	Low to medium	Medium	– –
Pizza	High	High	High	Medium	Low	– –
Cheese	High	High	Low	Low	Low	– –
Liver	High	High	Low	High, many vitamins	High	0
Egg yolk	High	Nil	Nil	Nil	Nil	–
Egg white	Nil	High	Nil	Nil	Nil	+
Poultry	Medium	High	Low	Low	Low	0
Fish	Low	High	Low	Low to medium	Low	+
Nuts	High	High	Medium	Variable	Low	0
Potatoes, bread, rice	Low	Very low	High	Low	Low	0
Spinach, greens	Nil	Very low	Low	High in B complex	High	+
Other vegetables	Very low	Very low	Low to medium	B complex vitamins	High	+
Oranges, citrus fruits	Nil	Very low	Medium	High in vitamin C	Low	+
Other fruits	Nil	Very low	Medium	Vitamin C, other vitamins	Low to medium	+

Minus signs indicate a negative effect and plus signs indicate a positive effect.

fatty acids, but most nuts, including peanuts, are fairly high in saturated fat content and hence bad for you. Next come milk products with high concentrations of fat, particularly cheese. Milk itself and yogurt also contain some saturated fats, but in lower concentrations. Low-fat yogurt is an improvement but still contains some fats and cholesterol.

Egg whites are made up of albumin, which is a near-perfect protein source, but the yellow yolk is pure cholesterol. I recommend chicken without the skin, which contains a lot of saturated fat. Fish not only has the advantage of high protein and low fat content, but some species like cod and halibut contain the "good" fats (including omega-3 fatty acids) and cholesterol, which may actually reduce the risk of heart disease and stroke. In fact, the fish-eating Japanese have one of the lowest rates of heart attacks in the world. So the old saying that fish is good for your heart and for your brain isn't too far off the mark.

Carbohydrates and Fiber

Carbohydrates are the body's main energy source, but if consumed in excess they are converted to fat and then deposited in all the wrong places. Bread, cereal, rice, pasta, and potatoes are foods that are rich in carbohydrates. For several reasons, vegetables and fruits are among the best types of food. They contain little to no fat, and their carbohydrate content is mainly glucose and fructose, simple sugars that are very easy to digest and convert into energy. Critically, they all contain a large quantity of fiber or roughage, which provides good protection against colon cancer and many other age-related diseases. Many of these fruits and vegetables contain vitamins and essential minerals, but the nutrient composition varies among different categories. Therefore, it is best to eat a wide range of fruits and vegetables.

Maintain Your Fluid Intake

Water is essential for life. But as we grow older, the brain's regulation of the thirst mechanism begins to waver, and it sometimes even forgets to signal that we should drink. Talk about a part of the brain itself having a poor memory! This can become a big problem for elderly people living alone, who easily become dehydrated, which in turn leads to severe medical complications and even death. Sound nutrition requires a daily fluid intake between thirty-six to sixty-four ounces (three to five glasses of water) daily; drink more in the summer and when you're exercising, less in the winter and when you're sedentary.

Vitamins: Diet Plus Supplements for a Promemory Effect

The beauty of vitamins is that they are completely natural substances essential for daily bodily functioning, and hence there is little danger in taking extra amounts, with a few exceptions. A diet rich in fruits and vegetables provides sufficient vitamins and minerals to prevent nutritional deficiencies, but a proactive intervention for memory loss requires supplementation well above the recommended FDA daily requirements. In other words, a healthy diet with proper nutrition is excellent for maintaining general health, but specific supplements are needed to obtain a promemory effect.

Destroyers of Free Radicals

The free radical theory of aging and memory loss lies behind the use of vitamin C and vitamin E, as well as vitamin A or beta-carotene. Vitamins A, D, E, and K are fat-soluble vitamins, whereas the B complex vitamins and vitamin C are water soluble. The fat-soluble vitamins are broken down mainly in the liver, which has a limited capacity to handle these compounds. Therefore, if taken in large amounts, fat-soluble vitamins like A and E can become toxic (vitamin D is needed for bone formation, and vitamin K is part of the normal blood-clotting process; these are not directly relevant to memory). In contrast, the water-soluble vitamins are essentially nontoxic because any excess is promptly flushed out by the kidneys into the urine. You need to understand this distinction if you are taking, or plan to take, massive doses of vitamins.

Foods Rich in Antioxidants

Broccoli	Blueberries, strawberries
Corn	Citrus fruits (oranges, grapefruit)
Beets	Plums
Carrots	Red grapes
Spinach	Kiwi
Red peppers	Peaches
Germs, seeds	Nuts

Vitamin A Is Good for Your Brain

Vitamin A is an antioxidant that neutralizes "bad" oxygen and shields the membranes of brain cells from injury. Research suggests that it may diminish the risk of heart attack and stroke (not yet fully proven) and thereby decrease the likelihood of memory loss. The nutritional supplement dose of vitamin A is 10,000 to 50,000 units daily, or 10,000 to 25,000 units daily when taken together with 15 mg of beta-carotene. Carrots are an excellent source of beta-carotene, which is closely related to vitamin A. While vitamin A doses up to 100,000 units daily are generally safe, megadoses of vitamin A can lead to liver toxicity. Vitamin A has antioxidant potency that is comparable to vitamin E, and hopefully it will be studied further in people with memory loss. Until then, vitamin A will remain a second-level intervention in the Memory Program.

Vitamin C: Was Linus Pauling Right after All?

Linus Pauling, who won two Nobel Prizes, began to be considered a quack after he advocated taking huge doses of vitamin C to fight the common cold and to tackle a host of other diseases. More recently, his original arguments have been vindicated as the free radical toxicity theory has taken hold. Vitamin C or ascorbic acid is an antioxidant and potent free radical scavenger, and may be able to block elements of the aging process, including memory loss. Oranges, grapefruit, berries of all types, grapes, and other citrus fruits contain lots of vitamin C, so deficiency of this vitamin is extremely rare. Many people supplement their diet with 1 to 5 grams of vitamin C daily, but its effect in preventing memory loss remains to be tested in a long-term clinical trial. Nevertheless, vitamin C's broad antiaging effects make it a useful component of the Memory Program. Its main side effect is increased stomach acidity and irritation.

Vitamin E: The Best-Studied Antioxidant

Among the antioxidants, vitamin E (alpha-tocopherol) has received the most attention. A study of Alzheimer's patients showed that 2,000 units of vitamin E taken daily was associated with a six- to nine-month delay in reaching functional end points such as taking care of personal hygiene or being placed in a nursing home. Vitamin E is now being tested in people with mild cognitive impairment, and it may have a positive effect on this group of people as well. My expectation is that the antioxidant properties of vitamin E will be even more helpful to those who have a good memory but wish to prevent future age-related memory loss. A daily dose of vitamin E is a central component of the Memory Program.

Vitamin E is known to boost T cell function, which is important for the proper functioning of the immune system, which defends the body against bacteria, viruses, and toxins. Vitamin E may also indirectly protect against heart disease and cancer. It is present in soybean oil, margarine, nuts, wheat germ, and seeds, but the amounts contained in these natural foods are insufficient to produce a strong antiaging or promemory effect. You need to take vitamin E capsules to get this added kick. The Alzheimer's study utilized 2,000 units of vitamin E daily, but this is a high dose that may increase the risk of bleeding, because vitamin E is an anticoagulant. Until systematic studies are conducted to compare different vitamin E doses in the prevention and treatment of memory loss, I suggest that you stick to a daily capsule of 800 units (400 units if you want to be more conservative). I myself follow this strategy.

Multivitamin Tablets

These are good for health generally; check labeling for amounts of specific vitamins contained in each tablet or capsule.

Vitamins C and E: separate supplementation well above daily FDA requirements is needed for a strong antioxidant effect as part of the Memory Program.

Trace Metals in Your Diet

Selenium is a trace element that has antioxidant properties and is claimed to be an antimemory-loss agent, but it has not been tested rigorously in people who have memory loss. There are other elements—magnesium and zinc in particular—that are necessary for normal brain function in small quantities, or traces. Until more solid evidence is forthcoming, and given the potential toxicity of these metallic elements and compounds, I don't recommend taking supplements of any trace metals. The amounts of these various substances present naturally in foods (and most multivitamin tablets) easily reach the FDA minimum daily requirement guidelines, so nutritional deficiency states are extremely rare.

Promemory Diet Action Steps
- Decrease intake of saturated fats such as red meat, pizza, desserts.

- Maintain your water and fluid (nonalcohol) intake.
- Eat fruits and vegetables, which are vital sources of antioxidants.
- Take a multivitamin tablet daily.
- Supplement with vitamin E and consider vitamins A and C as well.

Keep Exercising

Even very old people can benefit from a rigorous exercise program. Maria Fiatarone, a geriatrician at Tufts University, published a study in the *New England Journal of Medicine* in which a hundred frail, elderly nursing home residents (averaging eighty-seven years old) were randomized (equal chances of entering one treatment condition or another, like tossing a coin and seeing if it's heads or tails) to be in an exercise program that included progressive resistance weight training, intensive nutritional supplementation, a combination of the exercise program and nutritional supplementation, or a comparison (control) group that did not receive weight training. Compared to the control group, people in the exercise group more than doubled their leg strength in eight weeks. Perhaps even more important, nutritional supplementation alone did not do much good for physical strength and stamina, but the exercise plus nutritional supplementation group performed as well as the exercise only group.

The results of this study were striking, and the advantages of regular exercise are now universally accepted as part of any good health program, regardless of age. A recent study by Kramer and colleagues (1999) also produced impressive results: in 174 previously sedentary people sixty to seventy-five years old, regular walking led to improved performance on cognitive tests of executive function (memory was not systematically assessed in that study). As with diet, exercise should be a lifelong effort and not cease abruptly when you reach fifty or sixty or seventy. The body is a dynamic system and needs constant physical pruning and reshaping to perform optimally.

Physical Fitness Leads to Mental Fitness

In addition to its effects on the body, physical exercise also leads to "mental fitness"—improved cognitive performance, including memory. A clinical study showed that elderly people who completed a ten-week walking program showed significantly superior mood and

intellectual performance compared to another group of elderly subjects who continued their sedentary lifestyle. This effect has been confirmed in other studies that involved running and other strenuous
forms of exercise. But how does physical exercise work against memory loss? There are at least three possible explanations:

1. Effects on circulation in the brain.
2. Release of endorphins.
3. Impact on nerve cell branching within the brain.

Exercise Improves Your Circulation and Mood

Can exercise increase "brain tone" by improving blood circulation
and thus enhance memory? We know that regular exercise over a sus-
tained period of time can reduce the formation of cholesterol-rich
plaques that can block blood vessels, sometimes even dissolving
plaques that have already been formed, and thereby decrease the risk
of both heart attacks and strokes. Just as lack of exercise leads to fat
deposition and plaque formation in arteries, which can block blood
circulation, exactly the opposite process may occur when a sound
exercise regimen is implemented.

Describing a detailed daily exercise program is beyond the scope
of this book, but a few points are worth noting. Both aerobic and
anaerobic exercises are good for the heart and brain. Aerobic exercise involves medium-level effort in which the heart rate usually does
not rise by more than forty beats per minute. For most people, this
translates into a rise from 70 to approximately 110 beats per minute.
More severe exertion raises your heart rate even further and takes
you into the anaerobic range, when the body can no longer keep up
with the intensity of the exercise by utilizing glucose and has to switch
to a less efficient, anaerobic, energy-producing system. This is why we
cannot keep up anaerobic activity for long, and sprinting full tilt
beyond one or two hundred yards or meters is virtually impossible.
As you grow older, there is a good chance that you will choose to shift
from mixed aerobic-anaerobic (tennis, running) to purely aerobic
activity (walking, golf). Long, brisk walks are always a good form of
aerobic exercise.

After a good round of physical exercise, you feel exhausted. At
the same time, you feel energized, even a little high. This uplift is due
to the release of brain endorphins, which are chemicals that attach
themselves to opiate receptors, the same receptors that attract morphine and heroin. Endorphin release heightens attention and vigi-

lance, so your cognitive radar becomes a little sharper. This effect is short-lived, but regular exercise can prolong this effect.

Studies in animals show that exercise increases the availability of substances in the brain called neurotrophic factor and nerve growth factor, which stimulate the formation of new connections among nerve cells. Increased connections among nerve cells may indirectly protect against, or at least delay, degeneration of nerve cells during the aging process.

Regular physical exercise not only improves one's general feeling of well-being and quality of life, but it also has preventive and therapeutic properties against most of the major maladies that affect us as we grow older: heart disease, arthritis, and memory loss.

Exercise Action Steps for a Better Memory

- Perform moderate, regular exercise three to six times per week.
- Regulate aerobic and anaerobic exercises to your age, health, and tolerance level.
- Aerobic: brisk walking thirty minutes, jogging twenty-five minutes, swimming twenty minutes, formal exercise program in aerobics classes.
- Mixed aerobic and anaerobic: running, tennis, exercise equipment (stationary cycle, StairMaster, treadmill, NordicTrack, newer, low-impact workout machines).
- Before you lift weights, start with at least twenty minutes of aerobic or anaerobic cardiovascular fitness exercise (any of the options listed above).
- Yoga and related exercises are excellent for mobility but burn few calories.
- Keep a regular routine: don't overexert one week and become a couch potato the next.
- Stop if breathing difficulty or palpitations or faintness develops.

The bottom line is that proper diet and exercise make up the fundamental foundations of a sound program to prevent memory loss due to the aging process.

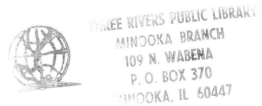

CHAPTER 6

Train Your Brain to Remember

Never Stop Learning

In the mid-1990s, a professor at one of my alma maters, the National Institute of Mental Health and Neurosciences in Bangalore, India, planted himself at my doorstep in New York. He was on a trip to Rio de Janeiro for an international conference and had arranged an "essential, educational" detour in North America before proceeding south. During his stay with me, he observed various facets of our department at Columbia University in action. Before he left for Rio, he summarized his New York experience.

"Here in America, you people keep learning all the time. From your interns and residents all the way to your senior faculty at the top. In India, we are just as good as the people in the United States at the stage when we finish residency training, but we tend to stop learning after we get a permanent faculty position. Your learning curve is a straight line that keeps going up, whereas ours climbs early on but then slows down and completely levels off. That is why you have accomplished so much more than your former classmates, who were just as good as you were, until you left and came to the States."

I have taken the liberty of paraphrasing what he said to make his gruff and curt utterances more reader-friendly. But the kernel of truth in his brief monologue, which I must confess had escaped me despite my having trained and worked for many years in both countries, is very important. I now think of "compound learning" in the same way that I view compound interest in an investment portfolio. A 10 percent annual increment in knowledge does not merely double the effect of a 5 percent annual advance. An annual 5 percent knowledge gain leaves you with a 70 percent increase in knowledge after ten years, whereas an annual 10 percent gain leaves you with a 180 percent increase after ten years. For an annual 20 percent knowledge gain, the increase after ten years is approximately 420 percent, which is literally six times the 70 percent increase seen with a 5 percent annual growth rate. So you should view learning as a lifelong and continuous process, and not sit back and vegetate after reaching a permanent position.

A Cliché That Works for Your Brain
Use it or lose it.

How Education Affects Memory: Rosa's Story

Rosa Gonzalez, a sixty-four-year-old woman from the Dominican Republic, was brought by her daughter into our Memory Disorders Center for evaluation of her declining memory. Rosa Gonzalez had forgotten to turn off the stove on one occasion and had begun to forget the names of distant relatives. Otherwise, she was functioning quite well at home, managing her daily chores without any difficulties. The neurological, psychiatric, and brain imaging workup revealed no significant abnormalities, but her neuropsychological test results threw us into a quandary. She scored in the range that would merit a diagnosis of dementia. However, her subpar scores were most prominent in naming, language, and general knowledge. She couldn't name any of the past five American presidents. From a set of ten pictures of objects, she couldn't name five: a camel, dominoes, a pretzel, a tennis racquet, and an igloo. On the Selective Reminding Test, which requires repeated learning and recall of a list of common nouns (like apple, chair, sky), she scored slightly below normal for someone of her age.

Rosa was tested in Spanish by a native Spanish-speaker. We expected Rosa to have difficulties in general knowledge and naming, because the tests are culturally biased against someone who did not grow up in the United States. However, tests of memory are more immune from cultural effects, and her below normal performance on the test requiring recall of a list of common nouns suggested a real deficit. Rosa Gonzalez supposedly had eight years of education, but on further discussion with her daughter it became clear that she'd had only four years of formal schooling.

Education is well known to have a major impact on performance for most cognitive tests, though less so for memory. I thought that this was probably age-related memory loss and not early dementia but wasn't sure. During the next four years, Rosa Gonzalez did not worsen in her neuropsychological test performance, confirming that she indeed did have memory loss due to aging and not a dementing process like Alzheimer's disease.

If You're Highly Educated, Subtle Memory Loss Is a Red Flag

This example shows that the impact of education (and culture) on cognitive test performance is almost as large as the effect of age itself. Education increases brain reserve capacity and thus decreases the likelihood of memory loss and intellectual decline. My colleague Dr. Yaakov Stern published a paper in the *Journal of the American Medical Association* demonstrating that highly educated people can mask memory loss by "talking around the problem" in the early stages of Alzheimer's disease. Presumably, their association cortex around the hippocampus is better developed, giving them a "cognitive reserve" that can be brought into play when the brain's frontline attempt at recall fails. So if you're highly educated, even subtle memory loss may be more serious than it seems, because it says that your strong cognitive reserve is breaking down.

The Kentucky Nuns Controversy

In a study of nuns residing in a convent, David Snowdon and his colleagues from the University of Lexington in Kentucky examined the autobiographical essays that all the candidate nuns were required to write when they joined the convent. The young nuns who had low "idea density" (number of ideas per every ten words) were significantly more likely to be diagnosed with Alzheimer's disease (diagnosed by brain autopsy) in their old age, compared to nuns who had written essays with high idea density when they joined the convent.

Does this mean that the template for developing Alzheimer's disease in old age is already set when we are young? We know that there is a strong genetic component to this disease, but for some reason it does not show up clinically until we are much older. Could it be that the educational process, and the additional mental challenges that galvanize us in many of our occupations, can stave off the illness for years, maybe even an extra decade? If that were true, it would represent one of the most intriguing interactions between genetics and environment.

But if you step back and think about this issue a little, you will recognize a few flaws in this tale. First, "idea density" is a poorly studied concept that does not directly follow from education or intelligence. Second, based on the results of the nuns study, the number of people with Alzheimer's disease should be far greater in underdeveloped countries with low levels of education and high levels of illiteracy, but cross-national studies show that this is definitely not the case. Stay tuned as further research helps to clarify this puzzle.

Techniques to Improve Your Memory

There are many books devoted to memory improvement by using a variety of tricks and techniques. I will not discuss techniques used by high school and college students to cram for exams, and instead will focus only on those methods that can help prevent age-related memory loss in people above the age of forty.

1. Pay attention. Pay attention to what needs to be learned or remembered. This seems obvious, but it's easy to lose track and forget things when you are pulled in many directions by personal or career demands. Reducing stress, and making a strong effort to maintain your concentration whenever necessary, are essential to improving your memory.
2. Heighten your sensory awareness. Heightened sensory awareness is essential to maintaining peak attention. Auditory memory makes use of the patterns, the rhythms of speech. Simple phrases, connected words that can be strung into a tune, these are techniques used by advertisers to zero in on your sensory awareness and get you to remember. The Nike, or Michael Jordan, phrase "Just do it!" is something most of

you will always remember, even if you have mild memory loss. Or the small elderly woman yelling, "Where's the beef?" in the hamburger ad. Three factors help imprint these memories in your brain:

    a. The dramatic nature of their content.

    b. The emotions they evoke in you.

    c. Frequent repetition that helps create a permanent auditory memory.

3. Be emotionally aware. Emotional awareness means being consciously aware of your emotions in relation to an event. Memories are registered best when the event has emotional meaning but doesn't overwhelm you with extreme anxiety or stress. This is why weddings and funerals are indelibly etched in our minds, yet there may be some parts that are simply not registered properly in memory because the emotions were too overwhelming. Focusing on the exact emotion you felt during the event will help you remember it better.

4. Focus to register a memory. Recognize the positive and negative influences that impact on your ability to remember.

Positive Influences	Negative Influences
Interest in the subject or event	Number of distracting stimuli
High attention and concentration	Dull content that evokes no emotion
Importance of the event in your life	Lack of familiarity with the event
The event occurs repeatedly	High stress level
Link to familiar things or themes	Depression or severe anxiety
Simple events are easier to recall	Poor health, experience of pain

5. Stay motivated. Scientists, athletes, writers, artists, computer scientists—they do not forget what they're supposed to do. Their motivation is so high that total concentration is a given, and the notion that they will lose track of what they're doing is unthinkable. In fact, on the rare occasion that it does occur—when a tennis star swings and completely misses the ball, or a baseball player takes his eye off the ball and makes an error in the field—we are surprised, even shocked. These maestros never forget their goal, and their focus is so strong that they can lose track of the passage of time.

And in your own life, when you are really enjoying a movie does your attention waver and lose track of what's happening? Of course not. You are so engrossed in the movie's details that forgetting isn't an issue. The same thing applies to reading a book that fascinates you. Motivation is what generates a high degree of concentration, and this leads to excellent recall of the event. But if you're not motivated to remember what you need to remember, here are a couple of tips:

a. Place the event in context to give it meaning. Focus on why you need to remember. Think about the positive aspects of the event and relate it to something else you like and know well. For example, if you're in a boring meeting, focus on someone you know or like in the room and link the points that you need to remember to imaginary actions carried out by this person.

b. Practice repetition. Even if you're not very motivated, repeating things in your mind will help you register the event. If you hear a piece of music often enough, and this includes music you don't really like, the tune will start playing in your head. That is how your hippocampus operates: if it receives a stimulus often enough, it gets registered as a piece of memory.

Mnemonics

The word *mnemonic* comes from the Greek goddess Mnemosyne, who knew everything: past, present, and future. Therefore, loosely translated, mnemonics can be used to remember almost anything. The memory questionnaire in the first chapter had a section on how frequently you use mnemonics.

In the loci technique, you create an imaginary house and place items you need to remember in specific rooms, using visual imagery. The peg technique involves the mental use of pegs or anchors for each event, and is similar to the loci technique. To work well, the loci and peg techniques require both an aptitude for visual memory as well as considerable mental effort. Teenagers and young adults are able to take advantage of these methods better than middle-aged or older people.

I will now discuss simpler mnemonics that include associations or links, rhyming and letter association, imagery and visualization, chunking, and lists and memory assistants.

Associations or Links

When you experience a new event, the hippocampus starts communicating with the parahippocampus, which is a big part of the neighboring "association cortex" in the brain, to see if the new event can be associated or linked with an older memory in storage. If it can be linked, the event is easier to remember and a new "memory link" is formed in the hippocampus and parahippocampus, which may in turn link up to even older memories stored in other parts of the temporal lobe or the frontal lobe. We all use associations or links, sometimes without even consciously knowing that it's happening. For example, some physical feature of a new person you meet, such as the eyes or forehead, can trigger a memory of a completely unrelated person who had similar eyes or forehead. This is a useless association because it doesn't help you in any way. On the other hand, linking a new acquaintance with another "memory storage" person with the same interests or in the same profession may give you a head start on dealing with this new acquaintance.

Create Interesting Associations

In its simplest form, creating an association or link is to connect the event you need to remember with something you already know. Another approach is to visualize and connect pieces of information into a story or action sequence. For example, if you need to take your dog for a walk, pick up your dry cleaning, and then call a friend, visualize your dog picking up your clothes between his teeth and handing them to your friend. If you are facile with language or have poetic ability, you can use letter or word links or rhyming associations to help you remember. If you are in the habit of doing this, you clearly prefer to tap into your auditory over your visual memory.

Visual Imagery

See it. People with a good visual memory can see things in their heads, and these memories stay long and firm in the hippocampus and frontal lobes, and can be retrieved later more easily. If you have this type of skill, you can use photographic or film techniques to boost your memory. The photographic technique is to consciously register each event as a photographic image in your brain, retaining all the elements as they actually occurred: the main person or centerpiece of the action plus all the surroundings. This strategy can be extended to the movie technique, because movies, after all, are a series of still images blending in sequence into one another. Some people have the ability to make up a story connecting various events and spin it into a movie sequence in their minds.

Visual imagery is much richer than verbal strategies where only the words are remembered and linked in some way. Unfortunately, only a minority of people have the aptitude, perhaps genetically inherited, to optimally use these visual imagery techniques.

How to Improve Your Memory for Names of People

How about remembering the names of people? This is what you need to do:

1. Pay attention.
2. Practice the name (repeat it silently).
3. Focus only on people you need or want to know.
4. Select one dominant feature of the person or event and link it with something or someone familiar in your mind.
5. Use other association links or images, if you wish.

How to Keep Track of Titles of Movies, Books, Authors

When reading a book or seeing a movie, we all start by registering the title or name in our minds, but then we get engrossed in the content of what we read or see, and the title begins to evaporate.

There are several methods you can use to improve your memory for titles or names:

- When you finish the book or the movie is over, make it a habit to spend an extra minute memorizing the title or name.
- You won't forget the main actor in a movie or the main character in a book, so another approach is to link the main character with the title by making up a little action-story in your mind.
- Using a link with something familiar works well. For example, I will never forget the movie *The Ice Storm* because it immediately

conjures up the stark beauty of a magnificent ice storm that I lived through in New Haven, Connecticut.

Like forgetting names, forgetting titles of movies or books by itself usually does not indicate that anything more serious is happening in your brain.

Chunking

Break up a large mass of information into smaller chunks under different subheadings to improve both learning and recall. Chunking is ideal for remembering numbers or a single, long sequence of information. It requires active conscious effort and practice, and is not as intuitive as forming associations or links.

Go Slow: Don't Try to Remember Everything All at Once

This dictum may seem self-evident, but many people do not recognize that the speed at which you can process information, more than the actual volume of data that can be handled by the brain, slows down considerably with age. An older person can learn the same amount as a younger person; it just takes longer, and this slowing down begins in middle age. This is because neuronal network data transfer has slowed down due to gradual decay of brain cells. So if you set unrealistic timetables for yourself that are based on your capabilities from twenty years ago, you increase the likelihood of failure. Pace yourself, because otherwise you may lose confidence and give up by thinking you cannot accomplish a task when, in fact, you can do it if you give yourself a little more time. This applies to both the speed of doing a specific task and the number of tasks that you expect to complete within a specified time period.

Organize, Organize, and Stay Organized

This is one area where aging actually confers an advantage; people above the age of forty are usually much better at getting organized and staying organized than teenagers or college students. This means that even if your hippocampal memory is not as good as it used to be, your "effective" memory in day-to-day living may actually improve as you utilize planning and organization to improve your executive skills and your ability to remember.

It is important to give yourself time to get organized. If you need to clear your head to get organized, lock your door, don't answer when someone knocks, and let the answering machine pick up your messages.

Keep Things in the Same Place

The trouble that many people have with finding their keys or purse or glasses can easily be avoided, especially at home, by being consistent about where they are placed. If you have to walk a few steps to return the keys or purse or glasses to their usual spot, the extra physical exertion is definitely worth it. Avoiding the mental aggravation that comes from trying to figure out where you might have misplaced an item is good for another reason: it decreases stress, and that is definitely good for your memory.

Planning: Pen and Paper Are Better Than Your Head

Planning is an integral part of getting organized. Spend the extra time you need to prepare for what you need to do before rushing headlong into it. Reducing your stress level will help you avoid making mistakes due to hasty action, be it at work, at home, or in the stock market.

Don't feel shy about using pen and paper! Notebooks (paper/pen or computerized) and lists are excellent memory aids. And if you suffer from moderate memory loss, you need to take this a step further: keep detailed lists and schedules, and paste important information in prominent places around the house.

Memory Helpers

Choose from this list of lists to suit your individual needs:

1. Daily planning list.
2. Weekly planning list.

3. If a list is too long, classify it into categories, for example, people to contact (call, E-mail), meetings to attend, business trips to make. A computerized word-processing or spreadsheet list is the best solution if many items need to be added and deleted frequently on an ongoing basis.

4. Calendars, appointment books, electronic organizers: make sure you refer to them after you actually make the entries. Stick with what makes you comfortable; the latest technology isn't the best for everyone.

5. You should carry your memory helper with you most of the time. Once you decide on what you will use, stick to it, don't lapse in keeping up. Periodically reevaluate whether you want to continue with it, for example, your appointment book may no longer be sufficient and so you might want to switch to an electronic device.

6. If you keep files in drawers and file cabinets, stick to your system and be regular in updating and checking your files.

7. If you use stickies for each piece of information, make sure you follow up and act on each stickie, then promptly destroy it to avoid stickie clutter.

8. Watch out if you're transferring information from one system to another, for example, handwritten notes to a computer document. This is where slipups often take place.

9. Be economical; don't use too many lists or types of lists. If you frequently discover that you don't remember what item you put down on which list, it means that you have too many lists and need to develop a new system that reduces the number or types of lists that you have.

In this context, I once had the misfortune of having a research coordinator (on one of my projects) who systematically wrote down every instruction on a notepad and then generated computerized list after list that she could never keep track of. This became a recipe for disaster—luckily minor disasters—until I insisted that she change her system and keep only one comprehensive computerized list that she updated regularly.

Trash the Junk

People who walk into my office are often shocked to see hardly any loose papers on my desk and conference table, especially those people who know how many clinical, research, teaching, and administrative balls I juggle simultaneously. My secret? When in doubt, throw it out! This is one motto that has stood me well over the years. I contrast this approach with that of some of my colleagues who keep wading through mountains of paper in their offices to try to find what they want; they always seem to be under stress and often cannot find what they want or need.

But what has this to do with memory? The fact is that you cannot hope to remember every little message, every small detail that bombards you every day. Clearing the debris in your mind is necessary in order to absorb and retain new information, just as you need to clean your desk regularly or clean out a house before you move in. So to keep your memory fit and ready to absorb new, important information, it is necessary to periodically extinguish useless lists, stickies, messages, stacks of papers, articles, and magazines.

Tips on Remembering Articles You Read, Talks You Listen To
What is the main point?
   Stay focused on this point (or a couple of points).
   Exclude the fluff, the unnecessary details.
   Get the gist, repeat it several times in your mind.

Age Does Matter

I strongly recommend the day-to-day memory aids and techniques described in this chapter, particularly if you are in your forties or fifties. Recent clinical studies have shown that if you're in your sixties to eighties, you may still experience positive effects but to a lesser degree than younger people. Regardless of your age, the effects will not be immediate and will be seen only after several months of practice, sometimes even years. While these methods are not a cure for age-related memory loss, they do form an integral and important component of the Memory Program.

Checklist of Methods to Improve Learning and Recall

Learning New Information	*Recalling Information*
Pay attention.	Go slow if you feel overwhelmed.
Increase sensory and emotional awareness.	Use associations and links.

Learning New Information	*Recalling Information*
Focus to register a memory.	Use visual imagery, letters, and rhymes.
Place the event in context.	Chunk numbers and parts of lists.
Consciously repeat it in your mind.	Organize: lists and memory helpers are essential.
Focus on the gist of what you see or hear.	Trash the junk; create memory storage space.

Above all, be positive about your ability to register new information and to remember it.

PART THREE

Prevent and Treat Common Causes of Memory Loss

CHAPTER 7

Mild Memory Loss: Fix Reversible Causes First

IT IS LIKELY THAT anywhere from 20 to 40 percent of cases of memory loss are due to specific, reversible causes. Therefore, if you suffer from mild memory loss, it is essential that you read this part covering potentially reversible causes of memory loss, because there is a distinct possibility that identifying and treating one or more of these factors will completely reverse your memory deficits. And even if you are not currently experiencing memory loss, you should be aware of the negative impact of factors like stress, alcohol abuse, depression, nutritional deficiencies, and hormonal changes on memory, so that you can reduce or eliminate their influence, both now and in the future.

A Case of Subtle Brain Toxicity: Jack's Story

Jack Kaufman, a tall, slim fifty-three-year-old bespectacled man living alone, came to see me in a state of considerable agitation. The previous week, he had lost the keys to his house and was forced to retrieve the duplicate keys from a neighbor, who luckily still had the extra set that Jack had entrusted to her. A few days later, Jack discovered that he had made a major error in his calculations for an office budget. He worked as an accountant and couldn't recall ever having made such a mistake. He said that his fear about losing his memory was disrupting his sleep, and that he could no longer concentrate on his work or his personal life.

I was a little surprised to see someone like Jack in our Memory Disorders Center. The episodes that he described could have happened to anyone, and most people wouldn't have rushed to seek help from a specialist. When I probed further, the source of his anxiety became clearer. His father had died of stroke, his mother from complications of Alzheimer's disease, and both conditions were present in the extended family on both sides. Jack's fears now made a little more sense.

Based on my interview, I determined that he had a very mild level of anxiety that did not meet diagnostic criteria for any psychiatric disorder. On neurologic examination, he had a generalized increase in deep tendon reflexes that could have been due to the presence of multiple small strokes in the brain. The MRI scan suggested the possibility of a very small stroke in the depths of the left frontal lobe, but the finding was so unclear that the radiologist hedged his bets and refused to call it a small stroke in his written report. I dredged up the scan from an obstinate medical records clerk and couldn't see any abnormality either (the radiologist was obviously much better at this than I, but it's a good idea for the patient's physician to also take a look). It seemed more likely that these abnormal reflexes, because they were widespread and not localized, were caused by heightened anxiety.

Neuropsychological testing produced a profile of no memory loss with mild deficits in attention and in the ability to change between "sets," which means that the rules of the test are changed in midstream and the subject is forced to readjust quickly and answer correctly according to the new rules. These deficits in "executive function" can be caused by a disease of the frontal lobe, that huge part of the brain sitting directly behind the forehead that is vital for intelligence and decision making, as well as storage of long-term memories. Sometimes, these frontal deficits are associated with specific neurological signs on physical examination, but these were totally absent in Jack's case. His performance could also have been caused by a lack of focus while doing the tests.

I wondered if his symptoms were all due to anxiety or if he had early signs of frontal lobe dementia, of which Pick's disease (microscopic structures called Pick's bodies are seen on brain autopsy) is one of the more common types. Or was he having ministrokes, which could give rise to a similar clinical picture, even though the MRI results did not clearly confirm this?

When in doubt, I usually do a few things. First, I talk to my neurologist and psychiatrist colleagues to see if they can give me some interesting leads, come up with a new idea, maybe dig up the files of another patient who presented similar symptoms. This approach didn't help me very much in Jack Kaufman's case. Second, I read the latest books and medical literature to see if they might shed light on the matter. This strategy didn't help me very much either. So I was beginning to consider my fallback position: recognize that I don't have the answer, discuss the situation with the patient, and explain that longer term follow-up with a trial-and-error treatment approach might be necessary.

But my curious diagnostic mind wasn't yet ready to accept defeat. Earlier, Jack had downplayed the impact of migraine headaches that occurred at a frequency of once or twice a month. On further investigation, he divulged the truth. Although the migraine attacks were not frequent, he often took painkillers as soon as he felt that an attack might be coming on. These included not only acetaminophen (regular Tylenol), but also Tylenol 3, which contains a small dose of codeine in addition to acetaminophen. Codeine is a narcotic that belongs to the same chemical class of substances as morphine and heroin, though it is much weaker in its effects. For most people, the codeine dose in Tylenol 3 is too small to have any impact on memory, but Jack sometimes took up to four tablets in a single day when he sensed the "aura" of an impending migraine attack. On days when the attacks did occur, he sometimes exceeded this dose.

Jack was unable to identify a clear time relationship between taking Tylenol 3 and his loss of memory, because his medication intake was erratic and unpredictable, which is why he hadn't reported it to me during the initial evaluation. I explained to him that there was a distinct possibility that the codeine in Tylenol 3 was having a subtle impact on his memory. Jack had obtained the prescription with multiple refills from an internist whom he saw barely once a year. Jack agreed with my recommendation to get an opinion from a headache specialist. The headache specialist stopped Tylenol 3 and switched him to sumatriptan (Imitrex), a powerful antimigraine medication that should be taken only just before or during a migraine attack, because frequent use is potentially risky. Jack had to adjust his approach to this new reality, but the great advantage was that when he took sumatriptan at the start of an attack, the migraine literally disappeared. Over the next few months, his cognitive abilities steadily improved, and he had no further incidents or episodes of memory failure. On repeat neuropsychological testing conducted a year later, he performed significantly better than he had when he first came to see me. We were both delighted with the result, and Jack expressed his heartfelt gratitude to me. He was now confident that he wasn't developing Alzheimer's disease or at risk for a stroke, but being a realist, he also knew that there was no guarantee he would be shielded from these conditions for the rest of his life.

Jack's story shows that it is often difficult to determine the exact cause of memory loss, but that persistence sometimes pays off. A few guidelines can help pigeonhole the symptom of mild memory loss into one of the following broad categories:

1. Memory loss due to the aging process itself.
2. Potentially reversible memory loss caused by a specific abnormality (Jack Kaufman).
3. Dementia, where Alzheimer's disease is the most common type.

If You've Developed Mild Memory Loss

- If you are in your forties to fifties, you are likely to have an identifiable, reversible cause of memory loss.
- If you are in your sixties to eighties, memory loss due to either the aging process or dementia is much more common.
- If there is a relatively rapid onset (weeks to months) of symptoms, a potentially reversible cause of memory loss is more likely.
- A fluctuating course of symptoms, with periods of clear memory and cognition intervening between episodes of confusion or memory loss, is more likely to be due to an identifiable, reversible cause.
- A gradual dwindling in memory over many years, even decades, is characteristic of memory loss due to the aging process.
- A steady decline with mild symptoms progressing to severe symptoms of memory loss within a few years suggests Alzheimer's disease.

The Aging Process Worsens Reversible Causes of Memory Loss

Some people with chronic depression or low-level medication toxicity develop mild memory loss for the first time in their sixties and seventies. Many of these people chug along for years with minimal memory loss induced by a specific, reversible cause, like depression or medication toxicity, because it is too subtle to affect daily functioning. Then the process of age-related memory loss, which has been progressing slowly but steadily in the meantime, catches up and adds an extra wallop that leads to clear-cut memory loss. In other words, the two types of memory loss may each be very mild, but when added together they cross the threshold above which most people recognize the presence of memory loss.

Clearly, it can be risky to assume that subtle memory loss is always due to the "normal" aging process. As Jack Kaufman's story illustrates, medication toxicity is a common, often unrecognized cause of generalized cognitive decline, including memory loss. Medication toxicity is only one of the common causes of memory loss that can be reversed by early recognition and intervention. Another example is when older people cannot recall what was said, because they suffer from a hearing loss. In these situations, the solution is a hearing aid, not treatment with memory-enhancing medications.

Identifying Reversible Causes of Memory Loss Is Critical

The importance of making sure that there is no potentially reversible cause of memory loss cannot be overemphasized. Just imagine taking a memory enhancer like ginkgo biloba or vitamin E when in fact the root cause is medication toxicity or alcohol abuse or depression or hormonal abnormalities. Not only will the memory-enhancing medication have no positive effect, but the fact that things do not improve will also mislead you into thinking that the memory loss must be the first sign of Alzheimer's disease. This can be disastrous, both emotionally and practically. Therefore, if you suffer from mild to moderate memory loss, do not automatically assume that you have age-related memory loss. Rather, you should examine your habits and daily routine to see if there might be an identifiable, potentially reversible, cause.

In the next few chapters you will learn about these specific causes of memory loss and the optimal therapeutic strategies to reverse them. I will focus on common disorders that frequently lead to memory loss, and will not discuss less common causes of memory loss, which include cancer (spread to the brain or general toxicity), multiple sclerosis, HIV infection, and Lyme disease. High fever and other conditions can cause acute memory loss as part of "delirium," but these illnesses tend to occur in hospitalized patients and are easily identified; hence they won't be discussed in this book.

CHAPTER 8

Stress and Depression

Both stress and depression can cause memory loss. They share one common feature: reduced attention and concentration with poor registration of the event or episode in the brain. As a result, the fragments that are recorded do not solidify into a piece of memory. Naturally, such a fragmented memory cannot be recalled accurately, and sometimes cannot be recalled at all.

The Stress-Memory Connection

A widely accepted definition of stress is that the demands you need to meet exceed your ability to perform them. While this definition does not cover all types of stress, it is simple and consistent with what most of us consider stressful in everyday life.

During periods of great stress we tend to make more mistakes than usual and don't remember things well, such as where we put our keys or tracking our appointment schedules. However, high stress levels do not always lead to memory loss. For example, most occupants of the White House have reveled in the challenge and have not broken down under the stress of all the responsibilities that are thrust upon them. Their stress is offset by the gratification that comes from the power, importance, and control in the presidential role. Also, these people have a great capacity to withstand and overcome stress, which is why they became successful politicians in the first place. At the opposite end of the spectrum, an employee performing boring, repetitive tasks—a postal worker is a prime example—may feel severely stressed because of monotony and lack of stimulation.

Most studies of stress have been conducted in young adults, usually undergraduate volunteers who earn a few dollars for experiments run by their professors. These studies show that if you are extremely anxious, performance on tests of cognition, including tests of memory, falters. At the other extreme, a very casual attitude totally devoid of nerves leads to an equally poor performance, probably because of lack of attention and focus. The best performance is produced if you are slightly anxious about doing well on the test but can still stay calm and think clearly while under the gun. To produce peak intellectual performance you need to focus and yet stay fairly cool, a combination that is not always easy to achieve.

When experiencing extreme emotional states, a person's recall can be quite different from what really happened at the time of the incident. Conflicts between family and friends are often precipitated by such highly emotion-laden events, and the warring parties may have completely different memories of the same incident. These contradictory memories lead to opposite viewpoints, which escalates the battle, because each side is convinced that the other side is lying outright or blatantly distorting the facts.

How does recall of an event become so far removed from the truth? The best explanation is that the nerve connections from the limbic system that convey emotional tone to a memory become so overwhelmed by the intensity of the emotions felt during the event that they either begin to misfire or are recorded inaccurately in the hippocampus, frontal lobe, and related regions. In other words, instead of the initial memory trace becoming accurately hardwired into long-term storage, the extreme emotional state drastically alters the course of nerve transmission and a distorted memory becomes hardwired in the brain. After this faulty memory is deposited in the brain bank, it becomes extremely difficult to change the individual's perception of what really happened, as I am sure you recognize from highly stressful episodes in your own life. The same process can occur in a court of law, where a witness who saw an event in a state of extreme emotion has inaccurate recall on the witness stand. This distortion may not be deliberate perjury but a direct result of the memory trace having been hardwired improperly into the witness's hippocampus and frontal lobes. Similar mechanisms can distort the recall of repressed memories of perceived, or real, sexual or physical abuse.

How Stress Affects Memory in the Brain

There are three biological theories of how stress leads to poor memory:

1. Corticosteroids cause damage to the hippocampus.
2. Chronic stress increases toxic free radical formation.
3. Stress stimulates the sympathetic nerves, which in turn leads to high blood pressure and heart disease, thereby increasing the risk of strokes in the brain.

The scientist Robert Sapolsky developed the first theory: excessive stress leads to increased production of corticosteroids, which inhibit the utilization of blood sugar, which in turn leads to death of nerve cells in the hippocampus. These provocative findings have convinced a whole slew of basic researchers to tackle this area of research, but the clinical data are not yet conclusive. Nonetheless, this theory suggests that the use of steroids, even when given for medically indicated conditions such as severe asthma, may not be very good for your brain.

Animal studies show that chronic stress can lead to increased formation of free radicals. As previously discussed, these free radicals, including "bad" oxygen, can inflict damage on vulnerable cells in the hippocampus and other brain regions. The outcome, not surprisingly, is memory loss.

There is a third, indirect, way in which stress can induce memory loss. Stress stimulates the sympathetic nerves that supply the heart and affect blood pressure. As a result, chronic stress increases the likelihood of heart disease and high blood pressure. High blood pressure and heart disease can, in turn, lead to the development of strokes, including ministrokes, in the brain that can affect memory.

So whichever way you look at it, high levels of stress are not good for your memory.

Reduce Stress Bit by Bit

The hallmark of successful stress reduction is to do it bit by bit, however small each element may seem, and keep at it on a continuous basis. The emotions attached to relationships, marriage, children, parents, and career can be overwhelming and make you feel that tackling the big problems in these areas is the only way to control stress. Unfortunately, solving these "biggies" is often very difficult and may be impossible to achieve; it is much easier to gain control over smaller sources of chronic stress. Learn how to relax, practice how to cut down the unnecessary stimuli in this era of information overload.

Action Steps to Reduce Stress

- Focus on reducing not only the big but also the small sources of stress. Try to mentally compartmentalize the stimuli that engulf you; focus on the immediate task at hand, one at a time.
- Constantly prune extraneous information to keep your life from being overloaded.
- Avoid conflict over trivial matters; let them drop.
- Be aware of the impact of high levels of anxiety, and emotional states more generally, in distorting the memory of specific events. This knowledge can help you deal with faulty memories (yours or others') that cause stress in close relationships.
- If you're in a boring job, seek other outlets and stimulating pastimes. If you don't have a hobby, start one.
- Avoid social isolation and maintain strong relationships: these factors are critical to prevent cognitive decline.
- When faced with high stress or anxiety, avoid overeating. If you're a frequent business traveler, watch out! A diet high in saturated fat accompanied by lack of exercise is bad news for both your heart and your brain.
- Keep regular bedtime hours; avoid alcohol and caffeine at least four hours before bedtime.
- Go back to the tried and true; whatever worked for you before in reducing stress will likely work again.
- A complete stress management program should also include other methods—yoga, meditation, prayer, and deep muscle or deep breathing relaxation, depending on your preferences.
- Talk about your problems; intimacy and sharing with your loved one or a friend often relieves stress. If this doesn't work, consider psychotherapy.

Social Isolation Leads to Stress and Memory Loss

Loss of loved ones, loneliness, lack of things to do after retirement, and health problems can be major sources of stress, particularly in older people, who may lose hope. As we all know, severe depression is common following the profound trauma of bereavement. What is less well known is that memory loss occurs during the grieving process. In my own experience, I had poor concentration with memory lapses for several weeks after my father's death. I lost track of what people told me at work and in my personal life, and I was functioning below par for quite a while. It was as if my brain was a sieve, with information not being registered properly for later recall because my mind was preoccupied with thoughts and emotions and scenes that involved my father and the rest of my family.

While many of these life events are unavoidable, maintaining an active social life can help prevent both mental and physical decline. You can get away with a solo existence when you are young, but such a lifestyle can become an albatross around your neck when you are older. Physiologically, social isolation leads to sensory deprivation and understimulation of brain centers, which in turn causes cognitive, including memory, impairment.

Insomnia

After reading that taking a brief nap in the middle of the day reduces stress and improves productivity, I've tried to implement this in my own work schedule, whenever possible. I must confess that I am unable to really nap in the required fashion, so what I do is put my legs up on a chair, close my eyes, concentrate on breathing slowly but steadily, and basically "veg out" for a few minutes. It definitely helps to reduce my stress level, keeps me refreshed for the rest of the day, and probably increases my productivity. Try this and see if it works for you as well.

Action Steps for Better Sleep
- Avoid alcohol late in the evening (at least four hours before bedtime).
- Avoid caffeine (coffee or tea) late in the evening.
- Keep a regular sleep schedule.
- Maintain a regular physical exercise routine.
- Bedtime rituals can help (not for babies only).
- Have a glass of milk (hot or cold) at bedtime. Milk contains the amino acid tryptophan, which induces sleep.
- If you fly across continents and get jet-lagged, several hours' exposure to sunlight (go out during the day) helps switch the sleep-wake cycle to the new time zone.

Insomnia commonly worsens stress and vice versa. Melatonin (discussed in a later chapter) or other over-the-counter sedatives should be considered only after the above approaches have been tried and have failed. If sleep difficulties persist for more than a few weeks, go see your doctor.

Depression and Memory

Depression is a common reversible cause of memory loss. Depressed people are often slow in their thought processes, and some find it difficult to retrieve memories. Depression causes a deficit in attention, and hence new information is not registered properly, so attempts at recall often fail because the external stimulus—meeting someone for the first time, for example—isn't recorded as a permanent memory in the brain. These two symptoms—slowing down of thought processes and poor attention—underlie memory loss in depression.

When Depression Strikes at Memory: Joan's Story

Joan Marciano, a fifty-six-year-old divorced woman living alone, walked slowly into my office and took her time sitting down. She worked in the casual wear section at a department store and said that she could no longer keep track of how clothes were organized in the various racks.

"I just can't seem to do my job. My memory is failing me," she said, straightening out a wrinkle in her navy blue skirt. "The young folks quietly help me out whenever I have a customer. Especially Maria, she's only twenty-one. I'm afraid that if Maria leaves, the others may not help me as much and I'll lose my job. And I'm barely getting by now, as it is."

She seemed listless and said that her physical energy was down. When I asked if she had ever been diagnosed or treated for depression, she was puzzled.

"I'm not sure what you mean by depression, doctor. I don't feel sad or blue. It's just a lack of feeling. I have no feelings at all."

This was a dead giveaway. Though we usually think of feeling sad or down or blue as being typical of clinical "major" depression, some depressed patients instead report a loss of all feelings in their lives.

An ambulance screamed outside our hospital, disrupting our conversation. Such sounds are par for the course in virtually every neighborhood in New York City. Joan lived in a quiet suburb in northern New Jersey, but she showed absolutely no reaction to the sound of the ambulance. She sat slumped in her chair, barely moving.

On further inquiry, she said that life was now a chore, the fun had disappeared. She couldn't concentrate on reading the newspaper, and was having trouble getting her act together to make it to work every morning. Her sleep was disturbed, but she still had a fair appetite and denied any physical complaints.

I realized that quick action was needed and immediately arranged for a number of tests to help clarify the situation. The medical diagnostic workup was within normal limits. On neuropsychological testing, she scored slightly below normal for her age on several measures of attention, concentration, and memory. Her test performance was confusing to the neuropsychologist, who could not decide between the diagnosis of depression and the early stages of Alzheimer's disease.

I was more confident about the clinical presentation. I made a diagnosis of major depression and asked Joan if she would agree to participate in one of my studies. The study involved twelve weeks of treatment with the antidepressant medication sertraline (Zoloft) to evaluate its effects on both depression and cognitive deficits in people who had both these problems. Joan was quite willing to do the research evaluation and interview procedures in the study, but she was reluctant to take medication, as many patients are. The situation was compounded by her insistence that she had a memory deficit, not depression, and so she did not want to take an antidepressant medication. I had to explain the relations between depression and memory loss in many different ways before she finally agreed to try the medication. I also told her that while the medication was likely to make her feel better, it wouldn't exert its full effect for a few weeks and so she needed to be patient. She wasn't, and skipped an appointment. Then she frantically called me to say that she had received an unfavorable report from her supervisor and was afraid that she would be fired from her job.

When she came to see me the next day, she remained ambivalent, even negative, about taking sertraline (Zoloft).

"I have to fight my problems without a crutch. I don't want to become dependent on this medication," she said.

I never cease to be amazed by the number of people who religiously take their medications for heart disease, blood pressure, or diabetes, usually for years without end, and yet refuse to take a medication to treat a disorder that is affecting their most vital organ, the brain. I decided to bring up this point as a tactic to get Joan to take her prescribed antidepressant medication.

"Please tell me something, Joan. You take Prilosec for your stomach problems. And you've been taking it every day for how many years? Five? Okay, five years. Now would you consider that a crutch? As being dependent on the medication?"

"No, well, that's different," she replied.

"How so?"

She paused, unable to give me a rational answer.

"You're not alone in this, Joan. A lot of people are willing to take medications for all kinds of illnesses, but when it comes to their own minds, it becomes a no-no. It's as if the stomach, or for that matter every other organ, is more important than the brain!"

She was taken aback, both by my tone and the content of my little speech. Her resolve began to waver, and I pressed forward. I warned her that her only hope to save her job was to follow through with antidepressant treatment, and after some hesitation, she agreed.

After one month on 100 mg of Zoloft, she had become more energetic, her memory was now fine, and she was no longer having any trouble at her job. In fact, she was effusively grateful and was so talkative that I became worried that the medication was flipping her from depression into mania, which is a syndrome characterized by the symptoms of hyperactivity with very fast speech, elation, grandiosity (statements like: I am unique, superior to everyone else), and impulsive, reckless behavior. I asked Joan if she would permit me to speak to her family or friends, and she gave me the telephone number of a close friend. Her friend informed me that Joan was now back to her old self, and that Joan's bubbly, outgoing personality had always helped her to be successful in sales. I was delighted that Joan wasn't cycling into mania. As part of the clinical study, a series of neuropsychological tests was repeated at the end of the twelve-week treatment trial. Her cognitive performance, including the results of memory tests, showed a marked improvement compared to how she had initially tested in the depths of her depression. This helped confirm my diagnosis of major depression, because a patient with dementia would not have shown this degree of cognitive improvement.

After the twelve weeks were over, on my recommendation she continued Zoloft for another year, after which I gradually tapered off the medication and eventually stopped it. Fortunately, Joan's depression did not return. She left treatment feeling happy, taking with her my instruction that she should call me if her depressive symptoms started to recur in the future.

How Depression Causes Memory Loss

Joan complained about memory loss even though her symptoms were caused by depression. In other words, memory loss masked her clinical depression, for which treatment was successful. Therefore, if you have begun to experience memory loss and you also feel down or blue (or lack all feelings) most of the time, depression may be the source of your memory problems. Depression itself may be related to stresses and traumatic events in your life, but sometimes depressive illness can strike for no apparent reason. This type of depression is likely to be due to abnormal chemical neurotransmission in the brain, which can be treated successfully with medications, as Joan Marciano discovered.

What If Memory Loss Persists after Depression Improves?

In some people with both depression and memory loss, the memory deficit may not improve even after the depression is successfully treated. In such a situation, the memory loss that accompanies depression may be the first sign of Alzheimer's disease. We showed this in a community study of 852 elderly subjects, where the presence of depression conferred a threefold increased risk of developing Alzheimer's disease during a follow-up period of up to five years. George Alexopoulos's research group at Cornell reported similar results in hospitalized patients who had both depression and cognitive deficits.

These results seem to run counter to the notion that memory loss is part of the depressive illness itself. The age distribution of the patients in Alexopoulos's and my studies provides a partial solution to this riddle. Our studies were conducted in people who were all more than sixty-five years old, with an average age in the seventy-five-to-eighty-year range. The findings probably do not apply to people in their forties and fifties, as illustrated by Joan Marciano's complete recovery from both depression and memory loss.

Diagnosing Depression

In the United States, the American Psychiatric Association's *Diagnostic and Statistical Manual* (*DSM*, version IV) is the standard diagnostic classification system for mental disorders. The *DSM* system divides depression into "major" and less severe categories. Major depression occurs in approximately 20 percent of people at least once during the course of their lifetimes, though at any single point in time only 1 to 2 percent of the population suffers from this condition.

DSM-IV Symptom Criteria for Major Depression

Major depression is indicated by the presence of either persistent depressed mood or pervasive lack of interest or pleasure in activities, accompanied by four or more of the following symptoms:

- loss of sleep or excessive sleep
- loss of appetite or excessive eating
- poor concentration
- excessive guilt
- suicidal thoughts or actions
- a feeling of hopelessness
- psychomotor (physical) retardation (slowing down) or agitation
- diurnal variation of mood (consistently feeling worse every morning or evening)

Most depressed people do not have such severe symptoms. Many people function moderately well but have always had a negative attitude toward life—the glass is always half empty. These people used to be classified as having "depressive personality" or "depressive neurosis," but now we think of them as having low-level forms of depressive illness that can respond to treatment. All of us can point to family members, friends, and coworkers who tend to be grouchy and grumpy—people with a negative approach to every task that they face. Their numbers have diminished in recent years, probably because many of them are taking antidepressant medications. In fact, in the mid-1990s, the *Wall Street Journal* ran a front-page article suggesting that widespread use of the antidepressant Prozac had led to less absenteeism and improved labor productivity in the United States. But if you're not depressed, these medications are not going to be of much help to you—unlike cocaine or amphetamine, they do not induce euphoria, and they are not addictive.

If You're Persistently Depressed, Get Treatment

Another issue is that as people grow older, there tends to be under-treatment of depression because many patients and physicians believe that depression is a normal reaction to the aging process. The argument against this belief is simple: if depression were indeed a normal part of the aging process, all the retirees in Florida and Arizona would be depressed and the beaches and golf courses would be empty year-round.

Antidepressant Medications

For depression of moderate to severe intensity (usually major depression), treatment with an antidepressant medication is required. The most widely prescribed antidepressant medications are the selective serotonin reuptake inhibitors, or SSRIs: fluoxetine (Prozac), sertraline (Zoloft), paroxetine (Paxil), and citalopram (Celexa), which work by increasing the availability of serotonin, a chemical neurotransmitter that seems to be deficient in the brain in many depressed patients.

The Truth about the Prozac Controversy

I am still astonished by how the media hype about Prozac has succeeded in misinforming depressed patients. The pro-Prozac crowd believes that it is a miracle drug. In reality, there is no basis for this notion. Scores of studies have shown that Prozac is as effective as, but not superior to, other antidepressant medications. The opposite myth, propagated by the anti-Prozac crowd, is that it is a highly dangerous and toxic drug. Nothing could be further from the truth. After the hue and cry about the possibility that Prozac may increase suicidal or homicidal behavior, the FDA carefully reviewed the available information from thousands of patients on this medication and concluded that the risk of either suicide or homicide was no greater with Prozac than with older antidepressants. The irony is that Prozac became popular precisely because it was non-toxic and easy to use, which is why so many primary care physicians prescribe it. More recently it has been claimed that long-term use of Prozac causes neurologic toxicity, and it remains to be seen if this is another myth that will be dispelled. Over twenty other FDA-approved antidepressant medications are also available. These prescription medications vary in their possible side effects, and require medical monitoring.

St. John's Wort and SAM-E

What about hypericum, otherwise known as St. John's wort? Many patients are already taking this agent when they first come to our depression clinic (I codirect both the Memory Disorders Center and the Late Life Depression Clinic at our hospital). Some people report minimal to mild improvement on St. John's wort, and others report no change whatsoever in their depression. The National Institute of Mental Health is now supporting a large-scale clinical trial to find out if St. John's wort really works. Another substance called S-adenosyl methionine (SAM-E) is also gaining popularity, but clinical studies with this substance have been very limited. More information from systematic studies is needed before I can recommend these alternative medications as treatments for depression.

Psychotherapy

Psychotherapy can be useful in the treatment of milder forms of depression. Cognitive-behavioral and interpersonal psychotherapy, which require the therapist to be very active compared to traditional psychoanalysis, have been shown to be effective in the treatment of mild to moderate depressive illness. Highly motivated patients show the greatest benefit from these forms of therapy—for example, cognitive therapy requires patients to do homework exercises to help correct their negative, distorted attitudes about themselves and other people. A recent pharmaceutical industry-supported study by Keller and his colleagues suggested a synergistic effect from combining the antidepressant nefazodone (Serzone) and cognitive-behavioral psychotherapy, but these results are not consistent with the prior literature on combining antidepressant medications and psychotherapy.

Action Steps to Prevent and Treat Depression

- Stress reduction (detailed earlier in this chapter) is good prevention.
- Maintain strong interpersonal relationships and social supports.
- If someone close to you says you're depressed, take the comment seriously and act on it because you may not recognize depression in yourself.
- Confide in family, friends, and religious advisers in whom you trust.
- If major depression is present, or if milder forms of depression last for more than several weeks, treatment with medications and/or psychotherapy is necessary.
- If you have recurrent depressive illness, the best prevention is to remain alert to identify the early signs of depression, such as dwindling interest in activities, feeling a little low, and sleep disturbance. If you recognize warning signs and symptoms based on your own experience during earlier depressive episodes, it is essential that you promptly seek treatment.

CHAPTER 9

Alcohol and Drugs

WITH AGING, ALCOHOL ABUSE continues to be common while other drug abuse declines. Yet because alcohol is considered socially acceptable, many people do not recognize its role in causing memory loss.

Early Signs of Alcoholism
- Do you drink every day?
- Has anyone ever told you that you drink too much?
- Do you tell family or friends that you drink less than you really do?
- Do you have gaps in recent memory, especially after drinking heavily?

If your answer to any of these questions is yes, and you suffer from memory loss, then alcohol becomes the prime suspect. During the aging process, the brain becomes much more sensitive to the effects of alcohol, as one of my patients illustrates.

"I've Always Had a Few Drinks at Night": Mary's Story

Mary O'Brien, a sturdy, jovial, sixty-four-year-old woman, complained of a gradually worsening memory over a three-year period. She lived with her husband and was close to her four grown children and nine grandchildren. I completed an extensive neurological, psychiatric, and neuropsychological evaluation that showed moderately severe deficits in recent memory associated with generalized brain atrophy on MRI scan. These results strongly suggested Alzheimer's disease. But as I usually do before I drop this diagnostic bombshell, I spent a little extra time double-checking all aspects of the patient's history.

I recalled that at her first visit, she had responded to the question about alcohol use by stating that she drank a little every day. After I received her alarming test results, I decided to probe further into this issue. Mary then revealed that she had four shots of whiskey every evening, a long-standing habit. Her husband confirmed her report. He also mentioned that she had begun to make up stories to fill the gaps in her recent memory, a tendency that is called "confabulation." Mary said that she had played with her grandchildren the previous weekend when in fact she hadn't seen them for a month. Confabulation is common in both Alzheimer's disease and Korsakoff's syndrome, which is the diagnostic term for a common type of alcohol-induced brain damage and memory loss. Heavy drinking damages the liver, which in turn causes thiamine (vitamin B1) deficiency. Thiamine is essential for proper utilization of glucose, which is the brain's main energy source. As a result, alcohol-induced thiamine deficiency causes damage to nerve cells in the hippocampus and two nearby structures called the amygdala and mammillary bodies that are also involved in memory processes. This leads to memory loss for recent events while most other intellectual abilities remain intact.

The neuropsychologist had concluded that Mary's test performance was consistent with a diagnosis of Alzheimer's disease, but her history of alcohol consumption made me think otherwise. So I decided to launch a systematic campaign to get Mary to stop drinking, or at least to reduce her alcohol consumption. Getting people to stop drinking or smoking is never an easy task, and these efforts are often doomed to fail. When I broached the subject, Mary fussed that there was nothing wrong in having a few "tonics" every day. After some thought, I realized that her husband, Sean, was the key. I spoke to him alone.

"Mary's four or five drinks a day are probably the cause of her memory loss," I said. "With age, her brain cannot handle the same amount of alcohol, which didn't create a problem when she was younger."

He paused to digest this new information. "I think I understand what you mean, doc," he ventured. "To tell you the truth, I was getting a little worried about that. But I can't get her to stop. She won't admit that she's drinking too much for her age."

"Does she drink alone? Or with you?" I asked.

"Oh, I have a coupla beers in the evening. Just to keep her company. Never more than a coupla beers. That's about it."

"I'd like to switch gears for a moment, Mr. O'Brien. You know the line about children doing what their parents do and not what their parents say?"

Sean O'Brien nodded with a quiet chuckle. "You're sayin' I've gotta stop first, right?"

"Exactly."

True to his word, he stopped drinking altogether. He also brought in a reinforcement; his oldest daughter joined the prohibition campaign against her mother. To my pleasant surprise, at her next visit Mary told me that she had cut back to two drinks a day. Sean confirmed that she had indeed reduced her alcohol intake. Eventually, she was able to stay off alcohol completely. Over time, her short-term memory gradually began to get better. During the following year, her memory showed modest further improvement, and during the next five years she maintained this performance level on tests of memory. Significant improvement in memory is virtually unknown in Alzheimer's disease, particularly over a prolonged period of time, while partial recovery after the patient stops drinking is typical of Korsakoff-type alcohol-brain syndrome. I was finally certain about the accuracy of my diagnosis.

Alcohol-Induced Brain Damage: A Clinical Chameleon

Mary O'Brien illustrates that steady, moderate- to high-volume alcohol consumption can affect your memory. But why some people are more vulnerable than others remains a bit of a mystery. Genetic factors can play an important role; people from a few Native American tribes are so genetically sensitive to alcohol that they can lose control and become violent after only one or two drinks. Clearly, psychological and social influences are also important.

More puzzling is alcohol's range of effects within the brain. Some people blithely consume vast quantities with no problems at all, some develop memory loss, others develop tremor and poor coordination because of damage to the cerebellum—a walnut-shaped structure in the lower, back part of the brain—and still others experience hallucinations. Research has taught us a great deal about the complex actions of alcohol at the molecular level, but we still don't know why such vastly different clinical disorders occur when people abuse the same substance in a similar fashion.

Tolerance and Withdrawal: Signs of Addiction

Tolerance means taking larger and larger amounts to produce the same pleasurable effects. Mary O'Brien was tolerant to the effects of four shots of whiskey every evening. However, this amount hadn't changed for decades, and she wasn't trying to increase her intake to get the same effect.

Alcohol withdrawal causes severe tremor, anxiety, sleeplessness, and occasionally hallucinations, together with severe craving for alcohol. Many alcoholics are terrified of reexperiencing these withdrawal symptoms and try to avoid them by never staying sober. Alcohol withdrawal symptoms require aggressive treatment, including hospitalization. Over the long term, many people benefit by joining Alcoholics Anonymous.

Warning

If you're depressed and also drink alcohol, your memory gets double-whammied.

Caffeine

Caffeine dilates the blood vessels and increases blood flow in the brain, which may explain why it seems to improve cognitive performance, at least in low doses. Caffeine also increases arousal and speeds up communication among nerve cells in the brain. This increase in alertness, a sense of being sharper, is what leads to better performance on cognitive tests, including tests of memory. But high doses can lead to adverse effects, including tolerance and even withdrawal, as any heavy user can testify.

On average, one cup of coffee contains the same amount of caffeine as three cups of tea. Caffeine is most commonly used to wake up in the morning, but some people drink coffee as a way to reduce stress. High doses of caffeine can lead to anxiety, jitteriness, and tremor of the hands. In other words, instead of reducing stress, caffeine can increase the sensation of being wired, resulting in difficulty concentrating and consequent memory loss. Therefore, as with many other substances, if you are a caffeine lover, moderation is the key.

Other Drug Abuse

Several illegal drugs—including marijuana, amphetamines, cocaine, and heroin—can damage brain functions, including memory. As with alcohol, the aging brain shows heightened sensitivity to most drugs of abuse, increasing the risk of memory loss.

Marijuana

Marijuana usually gives rise to a feeling of mild euphoria and a sensation of distance from the world that lies around the user. Although tolerance and withdrawal are milder than with alcohol, brain concentrations of cannabinoids, the active chemicals in marijuana, can reach astronomical levels.

Effects of Marijuana
- Interferes with acetylcholine production and thus lowers the level of this neurotransmitter that is important for attention and memory.
- High levels of cannabinoids in the brain lead to fluctuations in mental faculties, lethargy, and poor concentration, with inability to register new information and consequent memory loss.

People who quit using marijuana usually regain most of their cognitive abilities. In our Memory Disorders Center, we have seen patients in their fifties and sixties with mild memory loss who later improved when they discontinued the use of marijuana. These people had handled the drug with ease when they were young, but it finally caught up with them because the aging process in the brain made them more vulnerable to the drug's toxic effects.

Cocaine and Amphetamines

Cocaine ("crack" in its concentrated form) and amphetamines ("speed"; "Ecstasy") increase the release of catecholamines, a broad group of chemical neurotransmitters in the brain. Dopamine is a catecholamine that gives rise to the subjective sensation of pleasure and promotes adventuresome, novelty-seeking behavior. Not surprisingly, cocaine and amphetamines produce euphoria, a sense of being on top of the world, plus high levels of energy.

My Amphetamine Study

I once took a single dose of amphetamine as a "normal" subject in a placebo-controlled study (I was assigned to amphetamine, as I discovered later). Before taking the amphetamine, I did fairly well on a neuropsychological task in which unusual shapes rapidly flashed on the computer screen. According to the rules, I had to tap an electronic button whenever I decided that the flashing shape on the display had previously been shown to me. Without my knowledge, the complexity of the shapes that were presented were automatically adjusted on-line to keep me at an 80 percent accuracy rate throughout the testing period. Later, I found out that although I scored well, the computer easily boxed me into the 80 percent zone for accuracy.

But after I took the amphetamine, things changed dramatically. My performance became flawless and the computer could not keep up; I was getting everything right even though the computer was throwing all it could at me to try to drop my performance from 100 percent to 80 percent accuracy. The investigator conducting the experiment later told me that she had to discard my data because my 100 percent accuracy rate eclipsed the 80 percent upper limit permitted in the experiment. So my results could not be combined with those from all the other subjects who had stayed within the 80 percent accuracy paradigm set by the computer.

My performance wasn't related to learning the test, because the shapes were truly nonsensical, even bizarre, and kept changing continuously on the computer screen. Rather, after a single dose of amphetamine, the manner in which I processed information changed dramatically. Even though the time interval between the flashing shapes was only a second or two, I felt as if I had all the time in the world to think about each shape, decide if I had seen it before (memory processing), and then respond by hitting the button if I had. The speed of processing of new information in my brain—which in this study involved registering the shape and checking it against my memory data bank of recently viewed shapes before making the decision to give the command to my fingers to tap (or not to tap) the electronic button—was now so fast that the test itself seemed to have become slow. In fact, later that same day I asked if the presentation of the nonsensical shapes had been slowed down for me, and I was told bluntly that this had not occurred.

This is a well-known effect of not only amphetamines but also cocaine. Messages are transmitted and processed much faster by nerve cells, probably because of increased dopamine neurotransmission. This effect of amphetamines has been used by students to cram for exams at the last minute.

Toxic Effects: Psychosis

With both drugs, excessive dopamine release can cause psychosis with hallucinations (hearing and seeing things that are not there) and delusions (false, bizarre beliefs). Amphetamine-induced psychosis symptoms are similar to paranoid schizophrenia, while cocaine-induced psychosis is typically associated with grandiosity and the hallucination of bugs crawling on the skin. The psychiatric symptoms are paramount, and memory loss is secondary.

Narcotic Addiction

Narcotics were originally extracted as opium from poppies. Narcotics swing into action by attaching themselves to opiate (a type of chemical) receptors in the brain. Heroin, which is a first cousin of morphine, is the most addictive of this class of drugs. Even though some people get away with using heroin occasionally, for many others the addictive power is profound. Gene Hackman gave a terrifyingly accurate portrayal of heroin addiction and withdrawal in the movie *The French Connection*. Heroin is a central nervous system depressant and leads to lethargy, poor attention, and secondary memory loss.

Watch Out for Prescription Narcotics

Prescription narcotics like oxycodone (Percodan or Percocet) and codeine (Tylenol 3; remember Jack Kaufman's case in chapter 7) can produce a decline in many cognitive skills. The effects of these substances tend to be subtle, which is why most people who take them do not recognize their impact on memory. If you are taking one of these medications regularly and have begun to experience memory loss, check with your doctor for possible nonnarcotic options.

Tackling Drug-Induced Memory Loss Isn't Easy

With these various drugs of addiction, high doses often lead to amnesia, which is a technical term for memory loss. Being unable to recall, or only partially recall, the horrible subjective experiences when the drug's toxicity was at its peak makes it even more difficult for the addict to recognize the need to quit. Also, many addicts welcome drug-induced memory loss as a way to escape from life's problems, and this reinforces their desire to continue their drug use. But those who are able to kick the habit in time—alcohol and other addicting drugs alike—can regain all their intellectual abilities, including memory.

Stop the Addicting Drug and See If Memory Improves

If you, or someone close to you, are not sure if alcohol or another substance is causing subtle memory loss, there is a simple way to find out: stop taking the drug for two to three months and see if your memory improves. If it does, you have your answer, and staying off alcohol or the drug that you are using is the solution for your memory loss. But if you are unable to stop for even a few weeks, this proves that you are addicted and need to take specific steps, such as joining Alcoholics Anonymous or Narcotics Anonymous or another addiction program, to help you get over your addiction.

CHAPTER 10

Medication Toxicity, Infections, and Head Injury

MEDICATION TOXICITY IS A COMMON CAUSE of poor concentration and memory loss, particularly among people who take many medications. In this book, I generally give the pharmacologic name of the medication first, followed by the U.S. trade name (used to market the product) in parentheses, whenever applicable. For example, fluoxetine is marketed under the trade name Prozac, and acetaminophen is better known by its U.S. trade name Tylenol.

Signs of Medication Toxicity to the Brain
- Any sudden worsening in concentration or memory, or onset of confusion, after starting a new medication
- Any sudden worsening in concentration or memory, or onset of confusion, after a dose increase of an existing medication

Common Medication Culprits

Steroids, benzodiazepines, and medications with anticholinergic properties are among the commonly used medications that can cause memory loss.

Steroids

Steroids like hydrocortisone and prednisone are used to treat severe asthma and autoimmune diseases like rheumatoid arthritis and systemic lupus erythematosus (SLE or lupus). Many skin creams and ointments also contain steroids, but these are not absorbed in sufficient quantities to affect the brain. Steroids work by suppressing the body's natural immune response against bacteria, viruses, and toxins, and this helps in diseases where there is a wayward, self-destructive immune response. Steroids have a number of side effects, including stomach ulceration and weakening of bone structure (osteoporosis). In high doses, steroids can affect the brain, causing memory loss, confusion, and even psychosis. But subtle effects—particularly low-grade depression, anxiety, and memory loss—are far more common.

You may recall Sapolsky's theory that high levels of circulating steroids causing hippocampal neuronal loss lead to memory deficits, though whether this occurs clinically remains unclear. If you're on steroids and feel that your memory has begun to decline, report this symptom to your doctor, who may choose to stop the medication or lower the dose.

Benzodiazepines

Benzodiazepines comprise another class of medications that can cause subtle memory loss. From the 1960s to the 1980s, whenever patients seemed anxious or complained about sleeplessness, physicians routinely prescribed benzodiazepines. Over time, it became clear that benzodiazepines like diazepam (Valium) and flurazepam (Dalmane, "mother's helper" for sleep) had addictive properties. In the United States, many states have passed regulations that place benzodiazepines under the class of controlled substances, thus making them more difficult to prescribe. Nevertheless, most doctors still prescribe them, although on a more limited basis, because the other available antianxiety medications are not as effective.

Benzodiazepines can reduce concentration and cause mild memory loss. In elderly people, benzodiazepine use can lead to confusion, unsteady gait, and falls. Benzodiazepines need to be gradually tapered to reduce the risk of severe panic or seizures that can occur after sudden withdrawal.

Anticholinergic Medications

Acetylcholine is central to memory and attention, and it is present in high concentrations in the hippocampus and neighboring regions.

Therefore, medications with antiacetylcholine, or anticholinergic, properties can produce cognitive deficits that include memory loss. As with benzodiazepines, high doses can result in confusion and disorientation, though this occurs mainly in people who overdose. A variety of medications have anticholinergic properties, including older antidepressants like imipramine (Tofranil) and amitriptyline (Elavil), as well as antipsychotics like chlorpromazine (Thorazine), thioridazine (Mellaril), and olanzapine (Zyprexa). Acetylcholine also increases muscle activity and secretions in the gastrointestinal tract and bladder, so anticholinergics can cause the opposite: dry mouth, constipation, and urinary retention. As with steroids and benzodiazepines, if you're being prescribed an anticholinergic medication and have begun to experience memory loss, you should report this to your doctor and ask about stopping it or taking another type of medication.

Among the medications listed here, the research data on barbiturates, phenytoin, antidepressants with anticholinergic properties, benzodiazepines, narcotics, lithium, and cimetidine are fairly convincing, but there is less evidence to show that antihypertensives and digitalis cause significant cognitive deficits. Diphenhydramine (Benadryl), which is widely used, has antihistaminic and anticholinergic properties, both of which predispose people to cognitive impairment, including memory loss.

Dosage Makes a Big Difference

If you have memory loss and are taking one or more of the medications listed in the table, you should carefully review your situation. Keep in mind that most medication-induced brain toxicity usually occurs at moderate to high doses. Since almost all the medications listed in the table are prescription medications, you need to check with your doctor about the medication's impact on your memory.

If You're Taking Two or More of the Listed Medications
- The risk of memory loss increases.
- Ask your doctor if all the medications are really necessary.

Medication Rule
Don't stop or lower the dose of prescription medicines without checking with your doctor.

Medications That Can Cause Cognitive Decline, Including Memory Loss

Class of Medication	Names of Common Medications	Clinical Indication	Brain Toxicity in High Doses	Severity of Memory Loss
Barbiturates	phenobarbital Fiorinal (combination drug, includes barbiturates)	Seizure disorder, migraine	Widespread cognitive deficits	Moderate
Anticonvulsants	phenytoin (Dilantin)	Seizure disorder	Widespread cognitive deficits	Mild to moderate
Benzodiazepines	diazepam (Valium) flurazepam (Dalmane) lorazepam (Ativan)	Anxiety, insomnia	Poor concentration, memory loss, disorientation	Moderate
Anticholinergic antidepressants	amitriptyline (Elavil) imipramine (Tofranil)	Depression, also given for headache	Poor concentration, memory loss, disorientation	Moderate
Anticholinergics	Dramamine Meclizine Timolol (Timoptic) eye drops	Seasickness Glaucoma	Poor concentration, memory loss, disorientation	Mild to moderate
Steroids	prednisone cortisone	Autoimmune disorders	Depression, anxiety, psychosis, memory loss, confusion	Highly variable
Antipsychotics	chlorpromazine (Thorazine) thioridazine (Mellaril)	Psychotic illness, including schizophrenia	Poor concentration, memory loss	Mild
Lithium	lithium carbonate (Lithobid)	Manic-depressive illness	Widespread cognitive deficits	Mild to moderate
Narcotics	morphine oxycodone (Percodan, Percocet) codeine	Severe pain due to cancer, heart disease, arthritis	Widespread cognitive deficits	Mild to severe, depending on agent
Antihypertensives	propranolol (Inderal) methyldopa (Aldomet)	High blood pressure	Mild cognitive deficits	Minimal
Digitalis	digitalis (digoxin, Lanoxin)	Heart disease	Mild cognitive deficits	Minimal
Histamine-2 antagonists	cimetidine (Zantac) ranitidine (Tagamet)	Peptic ulcer disease, gastritis	Poor concentration, occasional memory loss	Minimal to mild
Antihistamines	diphenhydramine (Benadryl)	Hay fever, allergies	Poor concentration, memory loss	Minimal to mild

Manage Your Domestic Pharmacy

Maintain and update your domestic pharmacy on a regular basis, throwing away expired or unused medications. This roundup should include not only prescription medications but also over-the-counter and alternative remedies. As with prescription medications, some alternative medications contain substances that can be toxic, particularly heavy metals and anticholinergics. Since solid information on most alternative medications' brain toxicity is lacking, I have left them out of the table.

Environmental Chemical Damage to Your Brain Cells

Lead, mercury, arsenic, carbon monoxide, and organic solvents like benzene and toluene are toxic to the brain. Luckily, chemical exposure to large doses of toxins is largely a thing of the past, at least in the United States. Nonetheless, the problem does persist, since the control of auto emissions and industrial pollutants is far from perfect. Exposure to low levels of these toxins can cause mild cognitive deficits.

In children, nerve cells are still reproducing and growing, and heavy metals like lead wreak havoc on DNA and the process of cell reproduction. In adults, the nerve cells have already been fully formed, so the potential for brain damage and memory loss is much lower, though it still exists. In our Memory Disorders Center, we have seen a handful of middle-aged patients with possible heavy metal or organic solvent (benzene, toluene) toxicity, usually from a work-related source. In such cases, the facts can become a little murky if workmen's compensation claims are involved.

Carbon Monoxide Poisoning

Auto exhausts emit carbon monoxide gas, which atmospheric oxygen quickly converts to the less dangerous, though still unhealthy, carbon dioxide gas. People who try to commit suicide by carbon monoxide poisoning shut the garage doors to prevent access to fresh oxygen, connect the exhaust pipe to the interior of the car, and turn on the ignition. When this happens, the carbon monoxide from the exhaust competes with and displaces oxygen from hemoglobin in the body's bloodstream, thereby depriving vital tissues of life-giving oxygen. Therefore, the brain areas damaged by carbon monoxide poisoning are those that need oxygen the most: the basal ganglia that control motor movements and hippocampal nerve cells. Naturally, motor movement abnormalities and memory loss are common complications. If the person survives, the death of nerve cells leads to motor and cognitive deficits that neither improve nor deteriorate over time.

Infections

The formerly lethal bacterial infections of the central nervous system, particularly meningitis, are now invariably cured by antibiotics. Syphilis, which responds well in early stages to treatment with penicillin, is a sexually transmitted, bacterial disease that in its late stages can affect the brain. It used to be notorious for the chameleonlike quality of the different symptoms that it produced: unsteady gait, mood swings, psychosis, and memory loss. Some parasites can enter the brain and form a lesion that produces seizures and memory loss (though this is rare). Viral infections, including those caused by herpes simplex, can cause permanent scarring in the brain with cognitive deficits, including memory loss.

Prions are fragments of proteins and do not contain any DNA or RNA, which is the counterpart or mirror image of DNA. Because prions do not possess any DNA or RNA, they should not have life, which is defined according to the rules of modern biology as the ability to reproduce and propagate like viruses, bacteria, and the rest of the plant and animal kingdom. However, Stanley Prusiner, a recent Nobel laureate, has stuck steadfastly to the claim that these protein fragments can reproduce and cause diseases like Creutzfeldt-Jakob disease, a rapidly progressive form of dementia, and other slowly progressive neurologic disorders. The notorious "mad cow disease" is a close relative of Creutzfeldt-Jakob disease in humans, and may also be caused by prions. Some have begun to speculate that the elusive prion may also cause Alzheimer's disease. And I wonder, could prions play a role in memory loss due to the aging process?

Head Injury

The most common type of head injury is a concussion, which is external trauma to the skull (a knockout) without direct brain injury. A contusion is a direct penetrating injury to brain tissue and is much rarer. A history of head injury with loss of consciousness increases the risk of memory loss later in life, presumably by lowering the brain's cognitive reserve capacity against age-related memory loss.

Two widely quoted cases of structural brain damage have taught us a great deal about the seat of memory in the brain.

A Tamping Iron Went Through His Brain

Phineas Gage was a stalwart foreman working the railroad in Burlington, Vermont, in 1848. A misfired explosive blew a long tamping iron, which is like a crowbar, into his skull and through the other side. To everyone's astonishment, he was only stunned, got up, took a cart into town, and walked into a doctor's office for treatment. How could this be? The answer is simple. If the centers in the base of the brain (just above the neck) that control the heart and breathing are not affected, and there isn't undue mechanical pressure on other brain structures, the patient can indeed survive. Phineas Gage's injury affected the frontal lobes, and he developed a "disinhibition" syndrome with irritability and childlike capricious behavior that persisted for several decades after the injury. He constantly changed his plans and could not manage to complete even the simplest tasks. Despite the enormous size of his brain injury, many aspects of his memory remained fairly intact. This helped doctors realize that memory resides primarily in some region that was not destroyed by Gage's injury. However, the fact that he did have some deficits in recall showed that the frontal lobes are important, though perhaps not primary, for memory functions.

The Story of H.M.

This brings us to the 1950s and the story of H.M., who had surgical removal of large parts of both temporal lobes, including the hippocampus and neighboring amygdala, to treat uncontrollable epilepsy. His epileptic seizures stopped, but the cure may have been worse than the disease. He developed a profound defect in short-term or episodic memory, a type of severe amnesia. To this day, he cannot remember anything said to him barely a minute earlier, or recall having met a person a few moments ago. Remarkably, his recognition memory, which is distributed in many brain regions, including the frontal lobes, remains intact. Therefore, he can still choose the right answer, which he seems to have completely "forgotten," from a multiple-choice option. This startling discrepancy in his memory test performance is still difficult to explain fully, based on our current knowledge of memory processes. Nonetheless, his case, more than any other, helped to establish the hippocampus as the main seat of short-term memory in the brain.

Treating Memory Loss Due to Brain Damage

If infection or carbon monoxide or lead poisoning is caught early and the offending agent is treated or removed, there can be partial to complete recovery in cognitive abilities, including memory. However, if many nerve cells have already died, recovery may not be possible. In such cases, long-term physical and cognitive rehabilitation is necessary. Researchers are now trying various techniques to directly stimulate brain nerve cells to reproduce and replace those that have died, raising considerable hope for the treatment of such patients in the future.

CHAPTER 11

Hormonal and Nutritional Problems

Hᴏʀᴍᴏɴᴇꜱ ᴀʀᴇ ꜱᴜʙꜱᴛᴀɴᴄᴇꜱ ꜱᴇᴄʀᴇᴛᴇᴅ by glands without ducts, and they are transported in the blood to act at a special target organ or throughout the body.

The hypothalamus and/or pituitary gland in the base of the brain secrete their own hormones, such as thyroid stimulating hormone (TSH) or adrenocorticotrophic hormone (ACTH), to stimulate (or inhibit) the corresponding hormone-producing gland—for example, thyroid or adrenals (see Figure 2). This feedback loop is delicately balanced, and changes at either the top (hypothalamus or pituitary) or bottom (thyroid or adrenal) levels can lead to illness.

Diabetes Can Cause Memory Loss

Diabetes, which is caused by deficiency of the hormone insulin produced by the pancreas in the abdomen, leads to damage to very small blood vessels in different parts of the body, including the brain. Mini-ministrokes are the result, producing cognitive deficits that include memory loss.

Diabetes usually means high blood sugar or hyperglycemia, but the opposite—low blood sugar or hypoglycemia—can also occur because of overly aggressive insulin treatment or if someone takes insulin and then skips meals. Hypoglycemia is especially dangerous to the brain, which relies almost exclusively on glucose for its

111

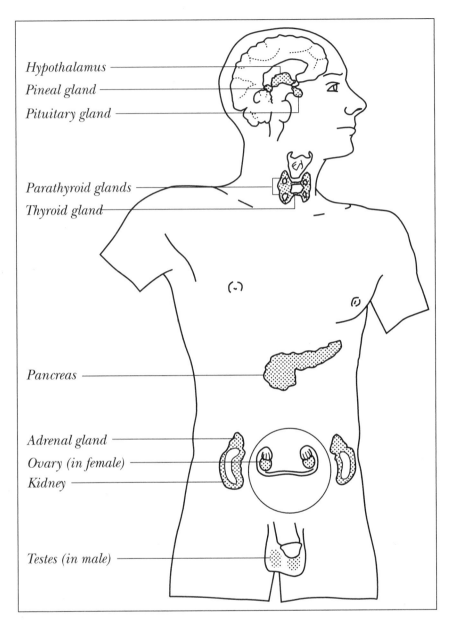

Figure 2. The main hormone-producing glands in the body.

nourishment. Hippocampal nerve cells have high metabolic needs and are very vulnerable to hypoglycemia; death of nerve cells with memory loss can result. Fortunately, most diabetic patients who maintain good control over their blood glucose levels do not experience this type of brain damage.

Thyroid Deficiency

The most common hormonal cause of memory loss is thyroid deficiency. A patient whom I saw early in the course of my career illustrates the effects of thyroid deficiency in the brain.

A Villager Misdiagnosed

After finishing medical school, I began my residency training at the National Institute of Mental Health and Neurosciences in Bangalore, India. I vividly remember the day in 1979 when a villager brought in his mother, Ponnamma. He stated that his mother had begun to hallucinate and talk to herself for no apparent reason, but he was a poor historian and could not specify if these symptoms were long-standing or recent. Ponnamma was obese and slow in her movements. I admitted her to the inpatient ward with the diagnosis of psychosis, a term that covers a broad range of severe mental illnesses, including schizophrenia. I ordered a set of blood and urine tests and started treatment with chlorpromazine (Thorazine), a medication commonly used to treat psychosis at that time. I went home quite pleased with the day's work.

The next morning, I received a stunning jolt. My senior resident, Dr. Raghuram, who had been on night call, summoned me into his office and lambasted me. Ponnamma had become nearly comatose during the night, and he had been urgently summoned to see her. After a quick examination, he correctly identified the physical features of obesity, slow movements, and absent reflexes as signs of classical myxedema caused by severe thyroid deficiency. He immediately started her on thyroid hormone replacement therapy. The blood test results, received the next day, confirmed the diagnosis. Ponnamma made a steady recovery on thyroid replacement and was discharged to her home four weeks later, free of psychosis and cognitive deficits.

This episode easily qualifies as the worst diagnostic mistake of my professional career, and the memory of that event is still crystal clear in my mind. The following year, I left the institute and emigrated to the United States. During my periodic visits to India, I make it a point to give a couple of lectures at my old institute and shoot the breeze with my former colleagues, including Raghuram. His clinical acumen, which helped straighten me out when I was a greenhorn, has been recognized and rewarded. He recently became the head of the department of psychiatry at the same institute.

"Myxedema madness" is caused by severe, prolonged thyroid deficiency, and is rarely seen these days because screening blood tests lead to early diagnosis and treatment. However, mild memory loss can result from mild to moderate forms of thyroid deficiency.

Symptoms of Hypothyroidism

Mental
- Depression
- Memory loss

Physical
- Weight gain
- Feeling tired, fatigued
- Puffy face and eyes
- Slowing of movements
- Drying and loss of hair
- Brittle nails
- Swollen neck (goiter)
- Intolerance for cold
- Constipation
- Slowing of heartbeat

From this list, if you have either depression or memory loss plus two or more physical symptoms, ask your doctor to check your thyroid hormone levels.

High Thyroid Levels

The flip side of hypothyroidism is the syndrome called thyrotoxicosis, which is due to excess circulating levels of thyroid hormone caused by autoimmune or malignant disease or by excessive hormone supplementation in people with thyroid deficiency. The clinical signs of thyrotoxicosis are hyperactivity, anxiety, and emotional instability. Memory loss can accompany poor attention and concentration resulting from the hyperactive state. Physical signs include heart palpitations, muscle weakness, and sleeplessness. For those receiving too much thyroid medication, the treatment is straightforward: lower the dose. For people with thyrotoxicosis due to autoimmune or other causes, there are effective antithyroid medications; surgical removal of part of the thyroid gland is occasionally needed.

Cushing's Disease

Cushing's disease is caused by excessive production of corticosteroids from the adrenal glands, which sit on top of the kidneys, and can cause memory loss similar to that caused by steroid treatment. Corticosteroids are important regulators of fat, protein, and carbohydrate metabolism, and Cushing's patients develop a "moon face" with considerable weight gain around the shoulders and trunk. Emotional volatility, anxiety, and depression are also seen in this condition.

What You Should Do about Hormone Abnormalities
- If you have symptoms that make you suspect hormone abnormalities, such as thyroid deficiency, go visit your doctor.
- If you receive any type of hormone replacement therapy and have begun to suffer from memory loss, report it to your doctor.

Nutritional Problems

When we think of nutritional deficiencies, malnutrition and starvation come to mind. But in the modern world of excess food production and consumption, the opposite type of nutritional abnormality predisposes people to memory loss. A diet rich in saturated fats promotes the formation of toxic free radicals in the brain. Equally important, cholesterol and saturated fats contribute to the formation of plaques that line the walls of arteries and smaller blood vessels, increasing the risk of stroke and cognitive deficits.

Niacin and Folic Acid Deficiency

In some cases, memory loss can be traced to vitamin deficiencies. The adverse effects of alcohol are partly caused by liver damage leading to deficiency of the vitamin B1, or thiamine, which is essential for the brain. Folic acid, or vitamin B7, deficiency is associated with anemia. Folic acid is known to help protect against colon cancer, birth defects in pregnancy, and possibly heart disease. Folic acid deficiency occurs in older people with poor diets, and can lead to memory loss.

Symptoms of Folic Acid Deficiency
- Lethargy
- Weakness

- Poor sleep
- Mild forgetfulness

Vitamin B12 Deficiency

Folic acid deficiency by itself does not cause severe memory loss. However, folic acid deficiency can aggravate the effects of vitamin B12 (cyanocobalamin) deficiency.

Symptoms and Signs of Vitamin B12 (Cyanocobalamin) Deficiency
- Deficits in touch, pain, and heat sensation
- Unsteadiness in walking
- Fatigue
- Memory loss
- Anemia (macrocytic type: large blood cells)
- Low vitamin B12 blood levels

If You're a Vegetarian

Vitamin B12 occurs only in animal products, so strict vegetarians are likely to develop B12 deficiency. But this standard medical explanation does not fit well with the facts: nearly a billion people in Asia practice strict vegetarianism for religious reasons, but their rates of vitamin B12 deficiency are no higher than in the United States or Europe.

There is another way to get B12 deficiency. A substance called intrinsic factor in the stomach is necessary for vitamin B12 to be absorbed into the bloodstream. So even if vitamin B12 oral intake is normal, lack of intrinsic factor in the stomach can lead to vitamin B12 deficiency. Special diagnostic tests help distinguish between these two causes. If there is intrinsic factor deficiency, swallowing more vitamin B12 doesn't do much good and monthly vitamin B12 injections become necessary.

If You're Older: Take a Daily Multivitamin Tablet

These vitamin deficiencies are rare but are becoming more widespread among the elderly who live alone or are disabled. They may not keep track of what they need to eat, or when they should eat. Problems with dentures also worsen nutritional deficiencies. Maintaining proper hydration and nutrition is essential. Family members who take interest, federally funded programs like Meals on Wheels, and the simple act of adding a multivitamin tablet to the daily diet are all useful and effective approaches that can prevent or reverse most of these nutritional deficiencies.

Hormones and Nutrition: Staying Well Tuned

Unfortunately, many people who develop memory loss assume that it must be due to the aging process and do not consider the possibility that reversible causes like hormonal and nutritional abnormalities may be the culprits. The good news about hormonal and nutritional abnormalities is that if they are recognized early, they usually improve and can often be completely reversed with the right treatment. For hormonal abnormalities, early recognition is the key and physician consultation is required. To prevent nutritional causes of memory loss, in addition to eating a diet low in saturated fats and rich in fruits and vegetables, taking a daily multivitamin tablet that meets the FDA requirements for the major vitamins (B1 to B12, A, C, D, E) is the best strategy. For a promemory effect, higher dose supplements of the antioxidant vitamins A, C, or E are necessary.

CHAPTER 12

Small Strokes, Big Strokes

Blockage of the arteries supplying the heart is the most notorious action of fatty plaques, but these cholesterol-filled growths occur just as often in the brain. There are many narrow, crooked, tortuous blood vessels in the brain, and these curves and kinks become the danger points: fatty, cholesterol-filled plaques stick to the inside walls and grow in size until they slow down blood flow, then a blood clot gradually forms and eventually causes complete blockage. When their blood supply is cut off, the nerve cells die due to lack of glucose and oxygen: this is the most common form of stroke.

Why Preventing Stroke Is So Important
1. Around 2 to 5 percent of people above the age of sixty will suffer a large stroke.
2. Small or ministrokes occur in 10 to 30 percent of people above age sixty. Most ministrokes occur without any symptoms ("silent" strokes) and are discovered only if a CT or MRI scan is done.
3. Each stroke, small or large, damages part of the brain permanently. Strokes occurring in the temporal or frontal lobes, or the pathways connecting them, often lead to memory loss.

Risk Factors for Stroke
- High blood pressure
- Heart disease

- High cholesterol
- Smoking
- Obesity
- Lack of exercise
- Diabetes
- Stress

Your preventive strategy should focus on reducing risk factors for stroke: reduce stress; go for annual medical checkups if you have a strong family history of stroke; reduce your weight and the intake of saturated fats in your diet; maintain regular exercise habits; take cholesterol-lowering medicines if proper diet and exercise together are not enough to keep your levels low; stop smoking; keep your blood pressure under control with a low-fat diet, low-salt intake, and if necessary, antihypertensive medications; and control diabetes (diet and/or medications) if you have this disease.

Three forms of cerebrovascular (brain blood vessels) disease can worsen cognition, including memory: transient ischemic attacks, ministrokes or small infarcts, and frank clinical strokes.

Transient Ischemic Attack: The Starting Point

A transient ischemic attack (TIA) involves partial blockage or spasm of a blood vessel in the brain without a complete cutoff in the blood supply. A TIA portends a stroke, just as chest pain due to angina warns of a heart attack. This is the stage where prevention and prophylactic treatment for a possible stroke are vital. If you have any of the risk factors for stroke, you need to learn a little about TIAs.

This Time, the Doctor Was Right: Joe's Story

My most dramatic patient with cerebrovascular disease had a TIA, not a stroke. In 1981, I was on night call as the emergency room physician when a man walked in with his wife. Joe Smith, a tall, massive construction worker in his late forties, said he had only a minor problem that needed to be checked out and didn't really feel the need to be in the emergency room. His wife, however, was very concerned and had dragged him to our ER under protest. The story that emerged started to ring alarm bells in my mind.

Joe had been doing an odd job in the house when he suddenly felt a tingling sensation in his right forearm and hand. He dropped his tools and stood up, then suddenly felt weak-kneed and had to sit down. After a minute, he felt fine, so he didn't tell his wife about the episode and resumed his handiwork. Half an hour later, the tingling sensation again ran down his right arm, and his right leg felt a little "funny." This time, he reported his symptoms to his wife. She noticed that he seemed a little confused and didn't remember what she had told him a few minutes earlier. She also knew that he was a stoic individual, and that he rarely complained about physical symptoms. Terrified, she brought him to the ER.

All his symptoms had vanished by the time they arrived. He was emphatic that he had never had any such symptoms before. He was a smoker and had a family history of heart disease, but no family history of stroke. His neurologic examination was completely normal. The history suggested a TIA, so I immediately paged the neurology resident on call. Enter Dr. Durocel, whose energy output greatly exceeded that of the battery bearing a close resemblance to his name.

After he heard my clinical presentation, his voice came through loud and clear, "Emergency CAT scan!" He quickly pushed the perplexed Joe into a horizontal position and charged with the stretcher toward Radiology. The technician performed at a speed that matched Durocel's, and within half an hour we had the CAT scan wet films. Joe had an aneurysm (ballooning of an artery) the size of a large peanut sitting on top of the left side of his brain. This aneurysm explained his right-sided TIA symptoms, because the left side of the brain controls the right half of the body, and vice versa. The location of the aneurysm on top of the frontal lobe also helped to explain his earlier transient confusion and memory lapses, because the frontal lobe plays an important role in long-term memory.

There was an imminent risk of aneurysm rupture and massive bleeding, which could be fatal, but Joe balked at the idea of brain surgery. Since his mild symptoms had disappeared, he was ready to pack up and go home. His wife was nonplused and a little paralyzed with fear. Durocel started screaming in frustration, and told the patient he was going to die if he didn't agree to surgery. This got Joe's back up even more, and I had to step in to calm things down. I took Durocel aside and suggested that we show the patient and his wife the CAT scan, where the aneurysm was clearly lit up in bright white against the gray-black of the cerebral cortex. As I had hoped, the dramatic image immediately caught Joe's and his wife's attention, and their mood began to change. After a few minutes of further discussion, Joe apprehensively signed on the dotted line for neurosurgery, which went without a hitch, and he was soon discharged home in excellent condition. Later, he wrote us a thank-you note, saying that he was back at work with no more problems.

Aneurysm Is Rare, Thrombosis Is Common

Aneurysms with the potential for bleeding are a relatively rare cause of TIAs, which is why I remember Joe's case so clearly. Most TIAs are due to cholesterol-laden plaques gradually blocking blood flow through a vessel; the TIA symptoms warn that the blockage is becoming severe and a clot or thrombus has begun to form. The clotting process is like a slow, relentless suicide machine: tiny particles called platelets in the blood begin to gather and aggregate to form a thrombus, the thrombus steadily mushrooms in size as more platelets land on it, and eventually the blood vessel is completely blocked. This results in an infarction (infarct), which is the death of a mass of brain tissue that is deprived of glucose and oxygen due to lack of blood supply. Nature has given us a powerful clotting process to shield us from excessive blood loss when we have an external injury, but the same process can be lethal if it occurs internally in the heart or brain.

> **Signs of a Transient Ischemic Attack (TIA)**
> **and What to Do When It Occurs**
> - Sudden weakness in any arm or leg.
> - Sudden changes in sensation (to touch, pain, or heat), speech, or vision.
> - Acute confusion or memory lapses that last for a few minutes to hours.
> - Any or all of these symptoms may resolve spontaneously, but this is no reason to rejoice. Go to your doctor or emergency room immediately, preferably accompanied by someone close to you.

Like Joe Smith, many people tend to wait because they usually recover without a hitch from the initial TIA, and when the full-blown stroke strikes it is often too late to treat effectively.

Types of Small and Large Strokes
- Thrombosis (clotting).
- Embolism (blood clot from the heart is propelled into the brain).
- Hemorrhage (bleeding, as from an aneurysm).

Embolism

I already described the mechanism behind clot or thrombus formation and the risk of hemorrhage (bleeding) from an aneurysm. An embolus is a thrombus that initially forms in the heart, often around a diseased heart valve. The thrombus is then mechanically dislodged and propelled by the heart's pumping action into the big carotid arteries going in a straight line to the head. The embolus flies through the wide carotids but then gets stuck in a slimmer branching artery inside the brain. The result, like a thrombus, is a stroke called an infarction or infarct. The embolus just sits there, blocking the blood vessel that used to supply the infarcting (dying) group of nerve cells in the brain.

Ministrokes

Ministrokes are usually caused by thrombosis, with clots forming in small sizes at different times from months to years apart. The death of nerve cells caused by each little infarct leads to a small degree of cognitive decline, including memory loss.

Typical Sequence of Symptoms
1. A sudden but small decline in mental faculties or slight weakness of an arm or leg.
2. Confusion and memory lapses that last a few days.
3. Gradual but incomplete recovery in mental faculties.

This sequence occurs because the brain reacts to the ministroke by pouring out edema fluid that compresses the area surrounding the dying brain tissue. As the edema subsides, the nerve cells that were compressed and paralyzed by the edema fluid regain their function, but those cells that already died in the center of the ministroke (infarct) cannot recover. Hence, there is only partial clinical recovery after each ministroke. If these little strokes occur repeatedly over several years, they can lead to full-blown dementia with severe memory loss. The history of repeated, staggered decline with incomplete cognitive recovery between episodes, together with clinical plus CT or MRI evidence of multiple strokes, help make the diagnosis.

Large Strokes

A large stroke is caused by blockage of a major blood vessel, most commonly the middle cerebral artery that supplies the regions of the brain controlling the motor and sensory systems, with loss of speech in the case of left-sided stroke. The middle cerebral artery supplies mainly the frontal and parietal lobes, and an area of the temporal lobe that does not include the hippocampus. Hence a large stroke causes only partial deficits in memory, primarily due to frontal lobe damage. These memory deficits can be difficult to assess in a patient with a paralytic stroke who has lost the ability to speak. Sometimes a large stroke can affect deeper parts of the brain, causing only partial paralysis, with speech being preserved.

Strokes, whether large or small, are most commonly due to a thrombus, less frequently an embolus, and rarely hemorrhage. This priority list of likely causes is the driving force behind current preventive and therapeutic strategies.

An Aspirin a Day?

Several studies involving thousands of people have shown that an aspirin a day reduces the risk of both strokes and heart attacks. This occurs because of aspirin's anticlotting (anticoagulant), not pain-killing, properties.

So after you make all the recommended lifestyle changes, the question remains: should you regularly take an aspirin (325 mg) a day? I advise you to take it daily as a good prevention for stroke, and even heart attacks, especially if you have one or more risk factors like a positive family history or high blood pressure or high cholesterol levels. You need to weigh this against the risk of stomach irritation and gastrointestinal bleeding; enteric-coated aspirin helps but not always. Some people take a baby aspirin (81 mg) daily, and this may be almost as good in doing the trick. However, if you don't have any risk factors for stroke, an aspirin a day is not essential.

Other Anticoagulant Medications to Prevent Stroke

For those who cannot tolerate aspirin, there are prescription medications such as Ticlopidine (Ticlid) and clopidogrel (Plavix), which

have similar anticlotting effects. Vitamin E also has anticlotting properties, but this is a weak effect that does not justify its use as a primary
stroke-prevention medication. Obviously, if you have a bleeding disorder, or are prone to excessive bleeding when cut or injured, you
should avoid these medications altogether.

Anticoagulants do a good job preventing thrombosis and
embolism, but what about bleeding or hemorrhage? Would hemorrhage get worse if an anticlotting medication were used? The answer
is yes. The same limitation applies to the use of powerful prescription
anticoagulants that are used to treat stroke in its early stages (or a
TIA). Heparin is injected acutely for this purpose, and oral warfarin
(Coumadin) is a longer-term anticlotting treatment. These anticoagulants are much stronger than aspirin and require frequent blood
tests to monitor the risk of excessive bleeding.

In recent years, a powerful anticoagulant with almost immediate
action, tissue plasminogen activator (TPA, Alteplase), has been developed. A single dose costs a fortune, but it can be effective in preventing the spread of a stroke in the brain after it has begun. The
diagnosis must be precise, because if a hemorrhage is misdiagnosed
as a thrombus or embolus, TPA can induce massive bleeding and even
death.

Steroids restrict the edema that follows a stroke, and are often
given as adjuncts to anticoagulants in the hospital. Acute stroke management is now handled like a heart attack, and the old rule that
nothing can be done to stop or reduce the size of a stroke once it has
begun is no longer true.

Stroke in its various forms is more common than Alzheimer's disease, and contributes to memory loss in a large number of people.
While you may think that your memory loss is caused by the aging
process, you may actually have been having ministrokes in the brain,
and accurate diagnosis with prevention and treatment can stop this
type of memory loss in its tracks.

CHAPTER 13

Alzheimer's Disease and Other Dementias

Some of you may fear getting Alzheimer's disease, and it is useful to know the basic facts about this illness. Also, understanding the boundaries between mild memory loss and Alzheimer's disease can help in developing your strategy to prevent memory loss.

Does Everyone Eventually Get Alzheimer's Disease?

Several years ago, Denis Evans's research group at Harvard conducted a survey in East Boston and found that literally half the people above the age of eighty met diagnostic criteria for Alzheimer's disease. Their results suggested that Alzheimer's disease, not memory loss due to aging, was the normal clinical course for people as they grew older. However, other investigators have since reported much lower rates of Alzheimer's disease in octogenarians. As I discussed in an earlier chapter, if performance on cognitive tests is corrected for age and education, then few people meet criteria for dementia, or Alzheimer's disease more specifically. But if absolute cutoff scores on cognitive tests are used to make the diagnosis without accounting for the impact of age or education, then a large proportion of elderly people will meet the diagnostic criteria for dementia, primarily Alzheimer's disease.

125

When Did Ronald Reagan's Alzheimer's Begin?

During a deposition in 1990, President Ronald Reagan could not recall the name of the chairman of the Joint Chiefs of Staff. We now know that he went on to develop Alzheimer's disease. Did he already have the disease at that time, or perhaps even earlier? While we will never know the answer definitively, his experience illustrates how Alzheimer's disease often starts. In Reagan's case it began with forgetting names, a common symptom of age-related memory loss. This is classic for Alzheimer's disease: in its very early phases, it is nearly impossible to distinguish it from memory loss solely due to the aging process, but over time, other symptoms develop. (Recall the case of Frieda Kohlberg, the seventy-four-year-old Holocaust survivor with a genius-level IQ whose only neuropsychological abnormality was a subtle deficit in recent memory; this was the first sign of Alzheimer's disease.) But with all the new technology now at our disposal, isn't there a better, more accurate way to make an early diagnosis of Alzheimer's disease?

Making an Early Diagnosis

The short answer is that no diagnostic test has been consistently proven to be better than a comprehensive neurological and psychiatric evaluation with careful history taking (increased age, low education are known risk factors), supplemented by a neuropsychological test battery, in making the diagnosis of Alzheimer's disease. The long answer is that there are many promising tests, each of which may have some clinical utility.

Early Diagnostic Tests for Alzheimer's Disease
1. After neurological and psychiatric evaluation, neuropsychological testing is essential.
2. Reduced ability to discriminate among smells (odors).
3. Hippocampal and parahippocampal atrophy on MRI scan.
4. Temporoparietal blood flow and metabolism deficits on SPECT or PET.
5. Decreased A-Beta protein amyloid and increased tau protein levels in the cerebrospinal fluid.
6. Presence of apolipoprotein E e4 genotype.

I will cover each of these in more detail.

Neuropsychological (Cognitive) Testing

Neuropsychological testing typically reveals that loss of recent memory is the only deficit in the disease's earliest clinical stages, which progresses over time to widespread memory loss, great difficulty in naming objects, poor fluency in reciting verbal material, and defects in constructional (drawing a cube, for example) and visuospatial abilities (finding the way to the neighborhood store). However, age and education strongly influence test scores, and these patterns of deficits can occur in conditions other than Alzheimer's disease. (Mary O'Brien, the steady alcohol user, was wrongly diagnosed with Alzheimer's disease based on neuropsychological testing.) The great strength of neuropsychological testing is its ability to pick up subtle, very early memory deficits.

Difficulty Identifying Smells

It sounds a bit strange: difficulty in identifying smells occurs early in the course of Alzheimer's disease. But there is a sound physiologic explanation: neurofibrillary tangles, a neuropathologic hallmark of Alzheimer's disease, infiltrate the "olfactory" or smell tract of nerve cells that goes from above the nose to a brain region just below the hippocampus. There are reliable standard tests of smell or olfaction that involve scratching a card and identifying the smell using a multiple-choice format. Our research group recently showed that the inability in people with mild memory loss to accurately identify smells strongly predicts who will later be diagnosed with Alzheimer's disease. Although the findings were strong, a number of factors can distort the results of the smell test: natural smelling ability varies markedly among people, smell discrimination skills diminish gradually with age, and smoking worsens smelling ability. So this test can provide a guideline but is by no means foolproof.

Brain Imaging in Early Diagnosis

In an earlier chapter, I discussed how an MRI scan can detect reduced size of the hippocampus and how SPECT and PET can detect reduced blood flow or metabolism in the parietal and temporal lobes. These features distinguish Alzheimer's patients from normal elderly people, but may not be as good in predicting who will get Alzheimer's in a group of people with mild memory loss. There are a few situations where these imaging procedures may be helpful—for example, a fifty-

year-old man with mild memory loss who shows the typical MRI and
SPECT/PET abnormalities is likely to be developing Alzheimer's disease.

Lumbar Puncture

A lumbar puncture is needed to examine the cerebrospinal fluid that
bathes the brain and spinal cord. Studies conducted mainly in Swe-
den, plus smaller American studies, show high levels of cerebrospinal
fluid tau protein (forms part of the neurofibrillary tangles) and low
levels of A-Beta amyloid protein (forms part of the amyloid plaque)
in Alzheimer's patients compared to normal elderly control subjects.
However, high levels of tau are also found in other neurologic conditions, so its diagnostic utility for Alzheimer's remains uncertain.

A few other diagnostic tests—a simple eye test, Alz-50 protein,
and the AD7Nc protein—were hyped up initially but fell by the wayside after subsequent research failed to replicate the original results.

Genetic Markers

Nearly half the patients with Alzheimer's disease have a family history
of dementia. Allen Roses, formerly the head of the Alzheimer's Center at Duke University and currently a division chief at the drug
company Glaxo-Wellcome, is the main proponent of using the
apolipoprotein E e4 genotype on chromosome 19 as an early diagnostic marker of Alzheimer's disease. However, not everyone with this type
of gene gets Alzheimer's disease, and some people who do not have
this gene can still get the disease. Also, there are big differences among
whites, African-Americans, and Hispanics in the risks associated with
this gene. Expert consensus panels have concluded that apolipoprotein E genotyping should not be used for clinical diagnosis.

Scientists have identified abnormal genes for a few rare forms of
Alzheimer's disease. Patients with abnormal presenilin 1 and presenilin 2 genes tend to develop Alzheimer's disease at a relatively young
age: forty to sixty years. There is one large family pedigree of Volga
Germans, now spread across the world, who provided the genetic
material that helped identify one of these genetic mutations. But even
in patients with early-onset disease, it is difficult to identify the presenilin 1 and 2 mutations because several dozen variations of each of
these two main mutations have been identified, and there probably
are many more waiting to be discovered. Therefore, complex laboratory techniques in specialized centers are necessary, and many

uncertainties still remain in using such techniques to make an accurate diagnosis.

The Clinical Picture Is More Important than Lab Tests

Once the initial hype settles down, the same issues tend to limit clinical applicability for all these tests: lack of specificity for Alzheimer's disease (which means that the same abnormalities are also seen in other diseases), uncertainty about whether they can be used at the stage of mild cognitive impairment to predict future Alzheimer's disease, and absence of replication in large-scale studies. If your doctor orders one of these (or other) tests, keep in mind that an abnormality on one of these tests does not necessarily mean you have Alzheimer's; the whole clinical picture needs to be taken into account before any diagnosis is made.

Progression of Alzheimer's Disease versus Age-Related Memory Loss

Alzheimer's disease is characterized by steady, progressive deterioration, with an average decline of 10 to 15 percent annually in memory test scores. Age-related memory loss is a different kettle of fish, and it is rare to see a decline of more than 1 to 4 percent annually in memory test scores.

Signs of Mild to Moderate (Early to Midstage) Alzheimer's Disease

- Frequently forgetting to turn off the stove.
- Getting lost when driving to a familiar place.
- Repeated mistakes in balancing checkbooks.
- Mistakes in executing familiar tasks at work or at home.
- Forgetting to get most of what was needed from the grocery store.
- Repeating the same phrases or sentences in conversation due to poor memory.

Coming to Terms with the Illness

Family members are often much more aware of the nature and likely course of the illness than the patient. This is because the dementing process often destroys the brain centers responsible for self-awareness, including the patient's own awareness of decline in intellectual capacity. Nonetheless, some family members refuse to accept that the patient indeed has a brain disease and get upset when he or she behaves in an irrational fashion. Coming to terms with the changing personality of the person they once knew is never an easy task.

Later stages of the illness are characterized by confusion and disorientation, inability to recognize family members, breakdown in the ability to manage bodily functions, and incontinence of urine. Some patients become mute, and psychosis and behavioral changes like agitation and aggression may occur. Managing patients in the final stages is virtually impossible at home, and admission to a nursing home or similar long-term care facility becomes necessary. For family members and close friends, the most disturbing turning point seems to be when the patient can no longer recognize them and has ceased to be the person whom they once knew and loved.

Potential Therapies

Caring for and treating patients with Alzheimer's disease costs over $100 billion annually in the United States alone. The introduction of FDA-approved cholinesterase inhibitors for treatment, and their potential utility in treating memory loss due to the aging process, has given rise to new hope that we are on the way to meaningful therapies for this terrible illness. There are suggestions that vitamin E, ginkgo biloba, estrogens, and anti-inflammatory agents may slow the progression of Alzheimer's disease, but some of these agents may be even more useful in preventing memory loss due to the aging process. I will discuss these therapies in the next major section in this book.

Other Dementias

Vascular Dementia

After Alzheimer's disease, the second most common form of dementia is vascular dementia, which is a direct result of multiple strokes destroying large portions of brain tissue (discussed in chapter 12).

Lewy Body Dementia

Diffuse Lewy body disease is a diagnosis that has gained in popularity in the 1990s. Lewy bodies are microscopic structures present in the brains of patients with Parkinson's disease. At least one-third of Alzheimer's patients also have clinical features of Parkinson's disease: tremor, slow movements, rigidity of muscles, and difficulty in walking. Some of these patients have Lewy bodies in addition to the typical Alzheimer's autopsy findings of neurofibrillary tangles and amyloid plaques. A British group headed by Ian McKeith has led the charge in calling for a separate diagnostic category called diffuse Lewy body disease, which has the clinical features of dementia, Parkinsonian signs, fluctuating memory loss and confusion, hallucinations, and extreme sensitivity to antipsychotic medications. Many cases previously called Alzheimer's are now called Lewy body disease; this topic remains controversial.

Frontotemporal Dementia

Frontal or frontotemporal dementia is a less common subtype. Earlier, all such cases were thought to have Pick's bodies, a specific type of microscopic abnormality, but many cases of frontotemporal dementia do not show this lesion. The clinical features overlap with those of Alzheimer's disease, but "frontal lobe disinhibition" signs are more prominent: overeating, sleeping excessively, hypersexuality, motor agitation, and impulsive and unpredictable behavior. Following damage to the temporal and frontal lobes, impulsive behaviors are unleashed from lower parts of the brain, as in the case of Phineas Gage, the railroad foreman whose frontal lobes were crushed by a tamping iron over a hundred years ago. For example, I remember a patient of mine with frontal lobe dementia who gained eighty pounds in one year and lost a hundred pounds in the next. These changes happened without any conscious effort on her part to either diet or put on weight. It was as if the appetite center in the hypothalamus (in a deep part of the brain) was receiving different inputs from the damaged frontal lobes in different calendar years. Some patients with frontal lobe dementia develop complete apathy and lethargy, a near vegetative existence. This can happen even when memory loss is only mild to moderate in severity.

Currently, there is no specific, approved treatment for either Lewy body disease or frontotemporal dementia.

Current Research Priorities

Making an early diagnosis and finding a treatment with robust effects are among the current research priorities in this field. If you already suffer from mild memory loss that continues to worsen even after you adopt the memory-enhancing strategies described in this book, I recommend physician consultation to make sure that you are not suffering from early dementia, whether it be Alzheimer's or a less common type.

PART FOUR

Medications That Prevent and Treat Memory Loss

CHAPTER 14

Medications: Regulated and Unregulated

Guilty until Proven Innocent

In a court of law, you are innocent until proven guilty. In science, you are guilty until proven innocent. The FDA assumes that medications don't work ("guilty") and that it's up to the pharmaceutical company, or whoever else is bringing the claim, to prove that the medication is more effective than placebo in a minimum of two separate double-blind (neither the patient nor doctor knows if active medication or placebo is given) clinical studies involving hundreds to even thousands of patients.

A Small Catch: The Practice Effect

As discussed in the Preface, in evaluating treatments for memory loss, a unique factor absolutely mandates a placebo-controlled trial. This is called the practice effect.

When you first try to complete neuropsychological tests, which include the tests of memory described in chapter 1, some parts seem difficult. The next time you do the same tests, you are likely to perform better, even on those tests that seemed hard to do the first time. This is the practice effect, which means that repeated testing results in superior performance because the brain automatically (even without conscious learning) begins to figure out how best to do the test. In people with little to no memory loss, the practice effect can last for many months after only a single testing session. Therefore, if neuropsychological test performance is compared before and after medication (or other) treatment for memory loss, there will often be some improvement due to the practice effect. If, however, active medication is compared to placebo, subtracting the change on placebo from the change on active medication gives us the real medication effect, thus accounting for the practice effect, which is assumed to be equal in people on active medication and people on placebo.

"I Don't Take Any Medications": Robert's Story

Robert Molson, a fifty-six-year-old man living in Greenwich Village, came to see me, stating that his memory had begun to decline, he was forgetting names more easily, and he was misplacing things more often. He was afraid he was getting Alzheimer's disease. He worked as a paralegal and hadn't yet run into problems at work, but he did point out that nothing short of a disastrous performance on his part would even be noticed in the New York City court system. He also had financial problems that were a source of constant worry.

He had no risk factors for dementia, and no neurological or psychiatric signs or symptoms on examination. I asked him if he was taking any medications.

"No," he replied bluntly.

Unfazed, I systematically went through a checklist of all possible medicines that people take for memory loss.

"Do you take ginkgo biloba?" I asked.

"Oh, ginkgo? That's a natural substance I get in a health food store; it's not a medicine," he stated categorically.

"Anything else you get regularly from a health food store?"

"I've tried ginseng a few times. And I take saw palmetto because I want to prevent prostate problems as I grow older," he explained. "And when I have a sleep problem, I sometimes take melatonin."

On neuropsychological testing, he performed very well. I reviewed the results with him, and he was relieved to learn that he did not have Alzheimer's disease. Since his main fear was resolved, he decided that there was no point in learning more about preventing age-related memory loss; that was the last I saw of him.

Many Natural or Alternative Remedies Are Also Medicines

Robert's most striking feature was that he did not consider ginkgo, ginseng, saw palmetto, or melatonin to be medicines. And because these were natural substances that he obtained in a health food store, he was willing to spend a fair amount of money on them despite his financial difficulties.

Many people do not count alternative remedies, or substances that occur naturally and are marketed for their health effects, as medicines. The reality is that many of these products do contain active ingredients, and the remedies that Robert was taking should be counted as medicines. Don't forget that many modern medications were first derived from naturally occurring substances, and the drug companies are always on the lookout for naturally occurring products with active ingredients that they can test against specific diseases. So don't take alternative medicines lightly; some of them do have active chemical compounds that have effects on various bodily organs, and some of them can cause side effects.

Regulating Alternative Medications

Alternative remedies, which are unregulated by any federal agency, have increased in popularity mainly based on anecdotal reports and beliefs: assume a therapy works unless someone can prove that it *does not work* (innocent until proven guilty). This approach is diametrically opposed to the scientific method underlying pharmaceutical testing and approval (guilty until proven innocent), and has created a bridge that has proven difficult to cross. Fortunately, the NIH has begun to fund randomized, double-blind, placebo-controlled clinical trials of these alternative remedies (NIH-funded studies of ginkgo for memory disorders and St. John's wort for depression are ongoing), to try to establish how effective they are and what side effects occur. Stay tuned for the results.

Worldwide Regulation of Medications

- Prescription medications are regulated strictly by the FDA in the United States, and over-the-counter medications are regulated to a lesser extent.

- Regulation of prescription medications is more lax in nearly all other countries compared to the United States. If a medication does not have major side effects, most European regulatory bodies will approve it as a prescription medication even if it hasn't been firmly proven to work in treating the illness.
- Alternative medications are not regulated by the FDA, but they are lightly regulated in a few countries.

These differences explain why a number of medications available in European and Latin American countries, including Mexico, are not available in the United States. Several medications that are approved in European countries—for example, nimodipine, which is used to treat vascular disease in the brain and is prescribed for dementia by many doctors—have failed to show superiority over placebo in American clinical studies conducted according to more stringent FDA standards. Germany regulates alternative medications, which places it a step ahead of the United States in this area. Talk of uniform international regulations has been making the rounds for decades, but no country has been willing to give up its prize turf in controlling the manufacture and flow of these money-making drugs. It is easier to generate a common Euro currency than to create a single regulatory body to approve new medications for all countries in the European Union.

FDA Does Not Approve Medications to Prevent Age-Related Memory Loss

The FDA does not recognize age-related memory loss to be an illness and is hence unwilling to approve any medication to prevent or treat this condition. This attitude has worked against research development efforts for both pharmaceutical agents and alternative remedies, because no company will invest tens of millions of dollars in clinical research on a compound or natural substance if at the end of this effort there is no hope of regulatory approval. This situation has led to most studies of new medications being conducted in patients with Alzheimer's, an FDA-recognized disease, rather than in people with mild memory loss.

Why Alternative Medications Vary in Quality and Content

The FDA requires pharmaceuticals, both prescription and over-the-counter, to be tested periodically to prove that their actual content lies within a 10 percent range of what is listed on the label: a 300 mg tablet must contain between 270 mg and 330 mg in serially tested batches, otherwise the manufacturer is forced to stop producing the medication. Such testing is not required for unregulated herbal, plant, or other alternative products sold in health food stores or similar outlets, which is why their content and quality, and hence their effectiveness and side effects, vary widely among different brands of the same product.

Taking Medications to Improve Memory: What to Ask Your Doctor

- Why am I taking this particular medication?
- How does this medication work on my memory?
- How much improvement can I reasonably expect?
- What is the right dose to take?
- Does it interfere with any other medicines I am taking?
- What are the common side effects?
- How long do I need to take it?
- Is the medicine addictive in any way?
- Can I drink alcohol while taking it?
- Is there any risk in stopping it for a few days at a time?

Most studies of treatments for mild memory loss have evaluated people over a few months or at most a year or two. If there is a slight improvement in memory functioning, will this effect be maintained ten, twenty years down the road? Also, will continuous long-term usage result in medication side effects that we did not see in the short-term? Although we don't yet have the answers from long-term therapeutic trials, the research evidence from short-term to intermediate-term studies with a variety of medications is now sufficient to help build a sound program to prevent memory loss due to the aging process.

CHAPTER 15

Alternative Remedies

FOR TWENTY-THREE YEARS, my father suffered from Parkinson's disease, a chronic, disabling brain disorder to which he eventually succumbed. Muhammad Ali, Janet Reno, and Michael J. Fox are among the prominent people who suffer from this illness. Parkinson's disease is caused by a deficiency of the neurotransmitter dopamine. The most widely used Western or "allopathic" treatment, Sinemet, is a combination of levodopa and carbidopa that works by increasing dopamine levels within the brain. This is by no means a perfect treatment, and at best staves off a few of the more nasty features of the illness. An episode that occurred early in the course of my father's illness helps to illustrate one facet of alternative medications in enhancing brain function.

A few years after my father developed Parkinson's disease, during one of my annual visits to my parents' house, I strolled in to see my mother in her bedroom. She was clad in a faded off-white sari, her domestic dress as per traditional custom. She sat cross-legged on the floor with two small mounds of silvery metallic powder laid out on a sprawling piece of paper. She was meticulously mixing the shiny substances together. She wasn't happy about my intrusion, and quickly tried to wrap up and hide the telltale material. I immediately guessed what was happening. In her frustration at the lack of response in my father's symptoms to Sinemet, she had turned to Ayurveda, the ancient art of medicine laid out in the encyclopedic Hindu texts, the Vedas. The shiny gleam in the metallic powder made me fear that toxic metals like mercury or lead might be hiding within. During my medical internship year in a rural setting in southern India, I had learned firsthand of the rapaciousness of fake Ayurvedic practitioners who thought nothing of adulterating historic remedies with their own brand of poison, purely for the sake of pocketing a few extra rupees. Heavy metal therapy is not unknown even in Western medicine, where injections of gold—yes, metallic gold— have been used successfully to treat severe rheumatoid arthritis. On the other hand, heavy metals can actually worsen Parkinson's disease, and I knew that Ayurveda had no effective treatment for this condition. I had a heated argument with my mother, and for a change, I won. She is well educated and knew about the toxicity of heavy metals like lead and mercury, but the tragedy of my father's illness had clouded her judgment and led her to desperately seek a remedy that might prove to be better than the standard medication, Sinemet.

The next example reveals the other side of the coin: an Ayurvedic preparation with potential promemory effects.

BR-16A: Travails of a Promemory Ayurvedic Preparation

A former colleague of mine, Dr. Chittaranjan Andrade, has studied an Ayurvedic preparation that now goes by its modern name, BR-16A. In controlled animal experiments, he showed that BR-16A improved learning and reversed short-term memory deficits in mice. But when he approached the four manufacturers of BR-16A in India, none of them were willing to fund further basic research to find out which of the twenty or more ingredients in the substance was responsible for improving memory. They also refused to fund controlled clinical studies in patients, because if one of the companies invested a large amount of money in research on BR-16A, any positive results obtained would translate into free profits for the other three manufacturers that had not invested in the research effort. As Chittaranjan discovered to his chagrin, it is virtually impossible to get financial support to conduct large-scale, systematic studies of Ayurvedic and other traditional medications. His basic science research on BR-16A is solid, and I think it is unfortunate that clinical development of this potential anti-memory-loss agent has been stopped in its tracks. "Memory-Plus," which contains the traditional medication "Brahmi," is also marketed in India, but the evidence supporting its use is much flimsier than with BR-16A.

Global Trade Practices

Many developing countries like India and China refuse to grant meaningful patent protection to drug companies because it is likely to raise the cost of prescription medications to levels far above the average person's ability to pay for them. Currently, the pharmaceutical industry in these and most developing countries consists mainly of chemical companies that copy and manufacture new medications developed by large multinational drug companies in the United States, Europe, and Japan. Only when countries like India and China finally pass meaningful patent laws will the clinical research floodgates open up in these nations, and we will then find out which of these traditional remedies really work for which disorders. Some of these traditional medications have been claimed to be effective against literally dozens of diseases, which is a little ridiculous. Systematic research is needed to find out which of these many claims is indeed valid. Unfortunately, the regulatory bodies in many developing countries have chosen to adopt an antiscientific approach in dealing with traditional medications. For example, the drug controller of India permits marketing of any medication that is described in ancient Indian writings and does not require any evidence whatsoever of either efficacy or safety of the traditional medication in treating a particular condition.

Keep an Open Mind about Alternative Medications
- Blanket support or disdain for the concept of "alternative" therapies is unwise.
- Alternative medications do contain chemical compounds, but they are derived from natural sources,unlike most pharmaceutical medications, which are manufactured.
- Some alternative medications are effective, a few are toxic and should not be used, and still others don't work but are generally harmless.

The Roots of Ayurveda

During my medical school years, I read some of the Ayurvedic texts, translated from Sanskrit into English, that described a wide range of therapies: herbs and plant extracts, metals, and bloodletting for various maladies. The vedas, among which Ayurveda is only a small component, were both the *Encyclopaedia Britannica* and the Bible of ancient Indian civilization. They were rooted in religion but contained a great deal of practical information and advice for everyday living. A number of Ayurvedic and related remedies have been "discovered" and subsequently used in Western medicine, including digitalis (digoxin) for congestive heart failure, rauwolfia alkaloids to extract reserpine (used to treat hypertension in the 1950s and 1960s), and several plant extracts with anticholinergic properties (to treat diarrhea, for example).

The Major Alternative Systems of Medicine

- Ayurveda is a complex system described in ancient Hindu religious and medical texts, detailing the use of literally hundreds of natural substances as medicines.
- Unani is a system of medicine developed centuries ago in Arabia and Persia, which later mingled with local influences in the Indian subcontinent. Its popularity has dwindled over time.
- Chinese medicines include a variety of plants and their extracts to treat both symptoms and diseases. Many of them are meant to promote health and block some of the effects of aging even in the absence of disease, and some of them have recently risen to prominence in the fight against age-related memory loss.
- Homeopathy originated in Germany two hundred years ago and has a worldwide following. Homeopathy relies on two principles: similars, and less is more. Similars refers to the theory that if a substance causes symptoms in a healthy person, the same substance in very small doses will cure a patient with those very symptoms. Less is more means that traces of active substances, usually mixed with sugar or other inactive substances, are sufficient to treat illnesses but are much less toxic than standard medications.

Proponents of homeopathy say that the minute dose of medicine has a powerful effect. The skeptical view is that the homeopathic sugar pill is no different from a placebo. But even if all that homeopathic therapy produced was a placebo effect, this is nothing to scoff at. Anywhere from 5 to 50 percent of people respond to placebo, depending on the condition being treated. As you might expect, a strong placebo response is virtually unknown in conditions like AIDS and cancer, but is fairly common in disorders like chronic back pain and depression. As I previously noted, the practice effect is responsible for a small, but highly consistent, improvement in memory on placebo, and this practice effect virtually mandates a placebo-controlled study. The main advantage of homeopathy, of course, is that because the tablets contain so little active ingredient it is usually harmless, which cannot always be said for the medicines from some of the older disciplines like Ayurveda and Unani. To my knowledge, there are no worthwhile promemory homeopathic medications.

Most of these older medical systems focused on the maladies of youth and middle age, because few people lived to a ripe old age in those times. Hence they had few medicines for age-related memory loss. The one exception: Chinese medicine, from which several remedies arose to treat the diseases of aging, including memory loss.

Ginkgo Biloba

Ginkgo biloba is taken by millions of people. As with many other organic plant extracts, anecdotal health claims abound for ginkgo. Many people think of it as a general tonic and consider memory enhancement as a sidelight. Others call it a fad that they wouldn't touch with a pole of any size. But what are the facts? What do we really know about ginkgo biloba?

Ginkgo contains many organic substances, which include flavonoids, terpenoids such as ginkgolides and bilobalide, and several acids. These ingredients have varying degrees of antioxidant activity, and this effect may underlie their promemory action.

Studies of Ginkgo Biloba for Memory Disorders

Nearly all the early studies that evaluated ginkgo biloba as a treatment for dementia came from Europe, and most did not employ rigorous research methodology. Then a North American consortium published a study in the *Journal of the American Medical Association,* utilizing EGb 761, an extract of ginkgo biloba marketed by a German company that provided the financial support for the experiment. In that study, of the 309 patients with dementia who were randomized to receive EGb 761 or placebo, only 78 patients on EGb and 59 patients on placebo were able to complete the one-year study. The EGb 761 study's results: even though the clinicians found no difference in their global impression between patients on ginkgo and placebo, patients on ginkgo showed significantly less decline on both a standard cognitive test and a forty-nine-item rating instrument completed by the caregiver (usually a family member). The test scores indicated that over the one-year study's duration, the ginkgo group held its own, with no cognitive deterioration. In contrast, the placebo group worsened appreciably. The magnitude of the effect was small (2 to 3 percent advantage for ginkgo over placebo on a cognitive test), which is probably why the clinicians' global impression showed no difference between the ginkgo and placebo groups. These findings are consistent with an earlier, less rigorous, study of 222 outpatients with dementia that showed 23 percent of patients improving on ginkgo biloba compared to 10 percent on placebo.

Side Effects of Ginkgo

In the EGb 761 study, other than a slight increase in stomach complaints, ginkgo's side-effect profile was essentially identical to placebo. But as with every medication, alternative or otherwise, ginkgo is not totally devoid of side effects. It has anticoagulant (anticlotting) properties that increase the risk of bleeding in the presence of other anticoagulant medications, particularly warfarin (Coumadin), which is commonly prescribed for people at high risk for heart attack or stroke. A few such cases of complications due to excessive bleeding have been reported in the medical literature.

Promemory Actions of Ginkgo
- Leaf extracts improve the ability of mice to remember newly learned behavior.
- In animal studies, enhances recovery from injury to the frontal lobes.
- In animal studies, acts against the memory deficits associated with aging.
- In a few clinical studies, slows memory decline in dementia.
- In healthy young adults, speeds up reaction time in stimulus-response tests, improving alertness.
- Anticoagulant properties may protect against stroke (and hence indirectly against memory loss).
- Antioxidant effects may protect directly against memory loss.

Ginkgo Improves Attention and Alertness

I have discovered that a surprisingly large number of people with mild memory deficits are taking ginkgo biloba. I have not yet seen a dramatic turnaround in any single individual, but some people do seem to become a little more alert. This may partly explain the results in clinical trials with ginkgo biloba, where the caregiver tends to report greater overall benefit than the clinician, who is focusing only on the memory deficit. Unfortunately, the studies with ginkgo have not used sophisticated neuropsychological testing to systematically evaluate the possibility that it leads to improved attention and greater alertness, rather than having a direct effect on memory. These activating effects may partly account for its promemory action: people who are alert and pay close attention tend to perform better on neuropsychological tests, including tests of memory.

Recently, a physician friend of mine told me that he now takes ginkgo regularly because he has a strong family history of Alzheimer's disease. And he definitely isn't the only card-carrying member of the American Medical Association who takes this substance. So even though the jury is still out, the evidence in favor of ginkgo is piling up to such an extent that former skeptics have begun to turn the corner. If you are worried about losing your memory, or have begun to experience subtle memory loss, or, as in the case of my friend, have a strong family history of dementia, ginkgo biloba is an option.

Ginkgo biloba is available in health food stores and no prescription is needed. Unfortunately, it comes in many shapes and forms, and you cannot always be sure of the quality of what you are buying. The *Journal of the American Medical Association* study was conducted with a ginkgo preparation called EGb 761 at a dose of 120 mg daily. This dose seems to be reasonable because it was associated with a mild positive effect in dementia while producing virtually no side effects.

If you decide to take ginkgo regularly, bear in mind that its promemory effects have been quite small in the studies conducted to date. Ginkgo biloba can play a useful role in a memory-loss-prevention program, but by itself it is unlikely to be the panacea, the magic potion, to prevent age-related memory loss.

Ginseng

Ginseng root preparations, used extensively in Chinese medicine for centuries, are now popular across Asia, Europe, and the United States. In the seventeenth and eighteenth centuries, its medicinal properties achieved such fame that fortunes were paid for prize roots, as if they were rare diamonds. The reasoning behind ginseng's use is that it repairs yang energy. It is believed to have broad antiaging effects and is often given to treat fatigue and impotence. Male rats fed on ginseng initiate sexual activity much faster than rats that do not receive ginseng.

Ginseng's Actions in the Brain

- Ginseng seems to increase mental alertness and then maintain it in a relatively steady state, thereby smoothing out the ups and downs of the stress response.

- Pharmacologically, ginseng may stimulate the production of epinephrine, which helps to indirectly suppress stress-induced release of cortisol and related steroids that may damage hippocampal nerve cells.

- Ginseng seems to boost cholinergic neurotransmission in the brain. Given the link between loss of cholinergic nerve cells and memory loss, this may explain its memory-enhancing effects.

- Ginseng contains a class of compounds called saponins, also known as glycosides, which may affect the function of neurotransmitters in ways that are not fully understood.

- In experiments involving people ranging from telegraph operators to students, ginseng reduces the time required to perform some neuropsychological tasks. This activating property may, in turn, lead to improved registration of new memories.

Types of Ginseng Preparations

Three common forms of ginseng are Asian (*Panax* ginseng), Siberian, and North American (*Panax quinquefolium*). The claims that any one type is superior have not been proven. Ginseng doses range from 500 to 3,000 mg daily, and the middle of this range is frequently used: 750 to 1,500 mg daily. A Chinese medicine called Ching Chun Bao contains a potent form of ginseng and is thought to be a general anti-aging tonic, juicing up energy level, sexual performance, and cognitive ability. Sometimes ginseng is marketed as a tincture that contains a fairly high alcohol content. People who take this tincture may feel better because of the alcohol and not the ginseng itself.

Given the limited knowledge base on ginseng in people with mild memory loss, I am currently not recommending it as part of your promemory program. The preparations listed above are not known to have any major side effects, so I am not campaigning against their use either.

Melatonin

Melatonin is a naturally occurring hormone that is formed mainly in the pineal gland. The pineal gland is the size of a small capsule and sits in the lower middle part of the brain. Descartes called the pineal gland the seat of the soul, but we now think of it merely as the source of melatonin, which regulates sleep and is involved in immune processes.

Melatonin for Sleep

Melatonin release from the pineal gland has a predictable twenty-four-hour cycle: an increase in the evening is associated with drowsiness and sleep, and a decrease in the morning leads to wakefulness. Melatonin production from the pineal gland declines steadily with age, and this produces disruption of internal clocks and rhythms, particularly the sleep-wake cycle. Melatonin is a good hypnotic, particularly for jet lag. I know a couple of physicians who work for the pharmaceutical industry, and they fly an average of once a week between Europe and the United States. They are quite happy with melatonin's effects in giving them a good six hours of sleep on the flight, and feel that it is a good antidote for jet lag. Melatonin doses of 0.5 to 3 mg are usually sufficient to induce sleep.

Melatonin for Memory Loss

Melatonin is an antioxidant, a superb scavenger of free radicals. Melatonin boosts its own antioxidant effect by promoting the activity of glutathione peroxidase, an enzyme that is also an antioxidant. Relatively high doses—3 to 20 mg daily—are taken for its antioxidant, and possible promemory, effects. Even in this higher dose range, it has few side effects. At doses above 100 mg daily, melatonin can do a reverse flip and cause insomnia and depression.

There have been many tall claims about the use of melatonin for a wide range of maladies, based primarily on results from animal studies. Clinical studies have focused on its sedative action, not its effects on memory. Its antioxidant activity suggests potential promemory effects. The lack of well-controlled studies using melatonin to treat mild memory loss or dementia, let alone to prevent memory loss, makes it difficult for me to recommend melatonin as a promemory agent. Also, I wonder if the anecdotal reports of melatonin's positive effects on memory are related to its property of inducing restful sleep and thus indirectly boosting daytime cognitive performance, rather than a direct memory-enhancing effect.

Alternative Brain Tonics

Coenzyme Q10 has been proposed as a brain tonic, but there are hardly any systematic studies with this compound. Other natural substances with possible promemory properties include gotu-kola, holly, calamus root, bhringaraj, and haritaki. Some of these traditional medications have been used for hundreds of years, while others are of more recent vintage. There are only anecdotal data to support their use as promemory agents.

Alternative Medications: Facts

- Among the current alternative medications, only ginkgo biloba has established cognitive-enhancing properties, though its effect is small in magnitude.
- You should consider taking 120 mg daily of EGb 761 (ginkgo biloba) as one of the medications in your memory program.
- More solid clinical evidence about the promemory properties of ginseng, melatonin, and other alternative agents is needed before they can be recommended for regular use.
- Phosphatidylserine (PS) is sold in health food stores. Some consider it to be an alternative medication because it is a naturally occurring substance, while others classify it as a pharmaceutical medication because an Italian drug company conducted the initial research with this compound. Phosphatidylserine is an important option in the Memory Program, and you will learn about its effects in a later chapter.

CHAPTER 16

Antioxidants

Vitamin E

A few years ago, a visiting speaker at our weekly departmental presentation praised the virtues of vitamin E as a potential treatment for several neurologic and psychiatric disorders, and as a general antiaging therapy. At the end of his talk, Dr. Jack Gorman, one of my colleagues who likes to occupy the front row, rose to his full height of six feet three inches and asked the speaker how much vitamin E he took daily. The speaker turned the question around and asked Jack how much *he* took daily. Jack immediately replied, "Four hundred international units." Jack is certainly not alone in this; many physicians, including yours truly, ingest a vitamin E capsule daily. In fact, the average daily dose of vitamin E has likely risen from 400 to 800 international units (IUs) daily among physicians, attesting to their growing faith in the antiaging properties of vitamin E.

Physicians Who Take Vitamin E

Doctors are notoriously bad patients, but they are often ahead of the curve when it comes to preserving their own health, as many are now doing with vitamin E. Remember how common it was for doctors to smoke in the 1950s and 1960s? At that time, many doctors were regular smokers in the United States, with even higher numbers in most other countries. But once the findings emerged on the links between smoking and both lung cancer and heart disease, many doctors quit smoking. Nowadays, barely 10 percent of physicians are regular smokers, the lowest proportion among the major professions. Similarly, while the number of overweight people keeps ballooning in the United States, physicians have reduced their own dietary intake of saturated fats. Physicians have finally become good at following their own advice, and statistics show that on average they live nearly five years longer than the rest of the population, despite constant exposure to infections and other diseases, long working hours, and high stress levels.

How Vitamin E Works
- Vitamin E is a free-radical scavenger that destroys toxic free radicals like "bad" oxygen and hydrogen peroxide; these antioxidant properties may benefit patients with Alzheimer's disease and protect against memory loss due to the aging process.
- The anticoagulant properties of vitamin E, which distinguish it from the other antioxidant vitamins A and C, may help protect against stroke.
- In laboratory experiments, exposing brain cells to vitamin E limits the number of cells damaged by glutamate, a naturally occurring substance that can act as a destructive neurotransmitter in many brain regions. This may be another method by which vitamin E protects against stroke.
- A Tufts University investigation found that a single 200 mg capsule of vitamin E daily significantly improved immune system response.

These broad antiaging effects of vitamin E have led to propositions that it can fight cancer, slow down the formation of cataracts in the eyes, and relieve arthritic symptoms. Some of these claims go way beyond the available evidence, and it remains to be seen if the actions of vitamin E are really that widespread.

Vitamin E for Memory Loss

In the Introduction, I described the story of David Finestone, a forty-nine-year-old man whose memory loss for names was probably caused by a small stroke. His treatment regimen consisted of cutting down on saturated fats, eating more fresh fruits and vegetables, taking an aspirin a day for its anticoagulant effects to prevent further strokes, and ingesting a capsule of 800 IUs of vitamin E daily. At that time, the antioxidant and antiaging properties of vitamin E were well known, but there were no data to indicate that it could directly prevent memory loss. However, recent studies have produced positive results, and vitamin E is now a frontline strategy to prevent memory loss due to the aging process.

Take Vitamin E to Prevent Memory Loss
- Vitamin E is present in high-fat (but luckily, low–saturated fat) foods like vegetable oils, germs, nuts, and seeds.
- It is impossible for you to get more than 200 IUs daily through diet alone.

Since vitamin E–rich foods can only go so far, you should take 400 to 800 IUs of vitamin E daily as a promemory (and antiaging, more broadly) dose, with 1,200 units for those among you who are more adventurous. Higher doses of vitamin E can cause headache, raise blood pressure, and increase the risk of bleeding in people taking anticoagulant medications like warfarin (Coumadin). There were few side effects in the study involving more than three hundred Alzheimer's patients who each took 2,000 IUs of vitamin E daily, but note that patients at high risk like those on Coumadin were excluded from study participation. Research-wise, large-scale, systematic studies with vitamin E have moved beyond Alzheimer's disease to people with mild memory loss, but these will take a few more years to complete.

The Antioxidant Selegiline or Deprenyl

Jozsef Knoll, a Hungarian university professor, developed selegiline as an antidepressant medication in the 1950s. Its antidepressant action is related to its ability to inhibit the enzyme monoamine oxidase-B (MAO-B), thereby raising the brain level of monoamines, which function as neurotransmitters. These monoamines include dopamine, which is needed for normal muscle control, sex drive, cognition, and novelty seeking or adventurous behavior. Based on its actions on the brain's dopamine system, selegiline is also widely used as a medication to treat Parkinson's disease.

Selegiline's Promemory Actions
- Inhibition of the enzyme monoamine oxidase-B, which in turn leads to a reduction in the formation of toxic free radicals.

- Stimulation of superoxide dismutase, a powerful naturally occurring enzyme in the body that also destroys free radicals.
- This dual antioxidant action likely underlies selegiline's action in delaying functional decline in Alzheimer's disease.
- Giving selegiline to mice leads to a higher density of nerve fibers in the frontal cortex and hippocampus.
- Mice given selegiline at about twenty-four months of age can increase, even double, their life expectancy beyond that point. In those studies, the mice demonstrated improved intelligence, measured by the ability to negotiate complex mazes and to develop a strategy to escape from water tanks. Experiments in dogs showed similar, but less robust, effects.

Obviously, taking selegiline will not double your life span as it can in mice, but its broad antiaging effects are a plus. Overall, the weight of the evidence suggests that it may be useful in preventing age-related memory loss.

Taking Selegiline to Prevent Memory Loss

Selegiline can cause insomnia, so it should be taken in the morning as a single daily dose. The usual dose range is 5 to 15 mg daily, though it can be given up to 60 mg per day to healthy people without any major side effects. Selegiline's action in inhibiting monoamine oxidase-B can make it toxic, but only in very high doses. Some physicians themselves use selegiline as an antiaging treatment. However, even among this group of people who can easily obtain medications, vitamin E is more popular. I have included selegiline as a second-level option in the Memory Program. Unlike vitamin E, selegiline is a prescription medication.

Vitamin E and Selegiline (Deprenyl)

My colleague Dr. Mary Sano headed a national consortium that compared four treatment conditions: vitamin E, selegiline (also called Deprenyl), vitamin E plus selegiline, and placebo to treat three hundred outpatients with early to midstage Alzheimer's disease. They found that both vitamin E 2,000 IUs daily (a high dose) and selegiline helped delay functional deterioration or nursing home placement by six months to a year. The results were published in the *New England Journal of Medicine* in 1997. Vitamin E alone, selegiline alone, and the combination of vitamin E and selegiline each delayed functional decline more than placebo. It was as if the antioxidant effect was "maxed out" by either compound, and hence adding them together did not improve matters any further.

Vitamin A

Vitamin A is essential for normal functioning of the retina, and its deficiency causes night blindness, which used to be fairly common until the latter half of the twentieth century. Beta-carotene is converted by the body's natural enzymes into vitamin A, and eating beta-carotene-rich foods like carrots prevents vitamin A deficiency. Both beta-carotene and vitamin A are antioxidants and free-radical scavengers, and many people take them regularly as antiaging medications. However, unlike vitamin E, vitamin A has not yet been tested against Alzheimer's disease or milder forms of memory loss.

Vitamin A: Doses and Side Effects

If you take vitamin A, your daily supplementation dose should be 10,000 to 50,000 units daily. Another option is to take 10,000 to 25,000 units of vitamin A together with 15 mg of beta-carotene daily. Vitamin A is fat soluble, meaning that if ingested in excess it cannot easily be flushed out by the kidneys like water-soluble vitamins (B complex and C), and it requires liver enzymes to detoxify the extra amount. Luckily, side effects occur only above 200,000 units daily, so the recommended therapeutic doses are safe.

Vitamin C: The Essential Acid

- Vitamin C (ascorbic acid) is essential for the nervous system, and is concentrated a hundred times more in the cerebrospinal fluid compared to other body fluids.
- Vitamin C is a strong antioxidant.
- In earlier times, sailors on long voyages deprived of citrus fruits (vitamin C) developed scurvy, a condition causing decay of skin and teeth.
- Older people who stop eating vitamin C–rich citrus fruits and vegetables may develop memory loss and mild confusion.
- At the opposite end of the age spectrum, students taking high doses of vitamin C tend to score slightly better on IQ tests.

Despite Linus Pauling's exhortation to swallow huge amounts of vitamin C to treat the common cold and other illnesses, clinical research in people with memory loss has been sparse. But given that it has antioxidant properties comparable to vitamin E, a promemory effect is more than likely.

Taking High Doses of Vitamin C Has Limitations

Vitamin C is found in most fruits and a few vegetables. I suggest a daily glass or two of orange or grapefruit juice, but if you want to be more aggressive you can add 1 to 5 grams of vitamin C tablets daily. Other than a possible increase in stomach acidity, you should not have any side effects. This is because as soon as the water-soluble vitamin C reaches high blood levels, the kidneys expel the excess into the urine. Effective therapy requires staying one step ahead of this mechanism, which means that unless you take high doses continuously, vitamin C therapy won't do you much good against memory loss. Another limitation is that vitamin C does not enter brain tissue easily. To cross cell membranes in the brain, fat-soluble forms of vitamin C like ascorbyl palmitate and ester C have been developed, but these medications have many side effects, and you should not take them on a daily basis.

Other Antioxidants

- Flavonoids, which are components of ginkgo biloba, are strong antioxidants.
- A subtype of flavonoids called proanthocynadin is found in grape seeds and pine bark. Grape seed extract and pine bark extract are marketed as antiaging products, but these substances have not been systematically studied.
- Green tea contains polyphenols that have antioxidant properties, and milk thistle extract contains the antioxidant silymarin.
- Barley and wheat juice contain large amounts of the enzyme superoxide dismutase, which is the main naturally occurring antioxidant enzyme in the human body.

For all these antioxidants, there isn't sufficient evidence for me to recommend them as part of the Memory Program.

Choosing Antioxidants to Prevent Memory Loss

The brain needs the same nutrients and vitamins as the rest of the body; it just needs a lot more of them. There is evidence supporting the use of antioxidants like vitamin E, and to a lesser extent vitamins A and C. One or more of these essential vitamins is a must in any program to prevent memory loss. One note of caution: these antioxidants are true long-term prevention agents and not quick-fix therapies. You will not see any immediate effects on your memory, and may not observe any change for several months. However, over a period of several years, there is a good chance that your memory will have declined less than that of your aging peers who have not chosen the antioxidant path. In any case, given that these are naturally occurring vitamins and related substances with hardly any side effects, and most are easy to obtain and not very expensive, what is the harm in taking them on a regular basis?

I am perfectly happy with my own regimen of lots of orange and grapefruit juice, which give me plenty of vitamin C, and a daily 800 IU capsule of vitamin E. Vitamin A reaches me as part of a multivitamin tablet, so I currently do not add specific beta-carotene or vitamin A supplementation. Right now, my memory is fine, but if for some reason I begin to develop any signs of memory loss, I may add vitamin A with or without beta-carotene. Similarly, I am holding off on using selegiline. But if you have already begun to experience mild memory loss, and you don't have an identifiable reversible cause, you could consider checking with your doctor about prescribing selegiline, in addition to taking vitamin E 800 to 1,200 IUs daily, with vitamin A or C as added options.

CHAPTER 17

Boosting Acetylcholine

Diane's Story

Diane Pozniak, a fifty-four-year-old divorced woman, worked during the day and took classes at night with the goal of obtaining a business degree and advancing her career and financial situation. She was not doing well in her classes and felt that it was because her memory was not good. She feared that these memory lapses would make it impossible for her to pass the required courses to complete her degree. On the other hand, she had no problems functioning at her day job as an administrative assistant. Her concern about memory loss arose from the fact that her mother had died of dementia in a nursing home, and Diane was worried that she had begun to get a similar illness.

On neuropsychological testing, she performed within the expected range for her age on most tests, except that her delayed recall score on the Selective Reminding Test, which evaluates the ability to learn lists of words and keep them in memory (a test described in chapter 1), was slightly below par. Her blood tests showed no metabolic, thyroid, or nutritional deficiencies, and her MRI scan was normal. Physically, she was in good health with nothing abnormal on her medical or neurologic examination. She seemed somewhat anxious and was clearly under stress, but I did not think she had an anxiety disorder or depressive illness.

I talked to her about her health habits, particularly the importance of reducing saturated fat in her diet and the need for regular exercise. She also listened to my advice about stress-reduction and relaxation techniques, but I had the distinct impression that she would not follow through with any action. She pointed out that she was so busy with a full-time job plus extensive schoolwork that she could not spare any time to go regularly to the gym, take walks, or start a stress-reduction program. She wanted a pill to help her memory, and after some thought, I advised her to start taking vitamin E 800 IUs daily.

She returned a month later in the same state, saying that she needed something stronger to help her because her performance in class had not changed despite her best efforts. She was convinced that this was solely because of her poor memory, and her earlier neuropsychological testing had suggested that this indeed might be the case. She was burning the midnight oil on a daily basis, so I knew her cognitive problems were not due to lack of effort. I decided to prescribe donepezil (Aricept) 5 mg daily.

A month later, she was grinning from ear to ear. She had just received a B in a class where just a few weeks earlier, she had fully expected to get a D or even an F. She felt more alert, and reported a distinct boost in her memory function. Out of curiosity, I repeated a few key elements from the neuropsychological test battery. There was some improvement in her performance on the Selective Reminding Test, but I could not entirely rule out a practice effect because she had done a similar test three months earlier. During the next year, she continued to maintain her improvement, and she successfully finished her business degree with above average grades. At no time was there a dramatic change in her cognitive test performance, indicating that the effect of Aricept was mild to moderate at best. But from Diane's perspective, it certainly did the trick.

Prescribing Off-Label Is Common

Donepezil (Aricept) is approved by the FDA for Alzheimer's disease, and not for the treatment of mild memory loss. So what on earth was I doing prescribing this medication to Diane Pozniak, who had very mild memory loss by any definition, someone who clearly did not have any signs of dementia or Alzheimer's disease? The answer to this seemingly loaded question is quite straightforward. Although the FDA "labels" the use of a medication only for a specific disease or diseases, all licensed physicians are free to prescribe approved medications for other conditions if they wish to do so. Obviously, if something goes wrong and a lawsuit ensues, the physician will have a tough time explaining off-label prescribing in court. In reality, many physicians, particularly psychiatrists and neurologists, prescribe medications off-label. This is because there is a wide gap between patients' needs and what the FDA has been willing to approve for a variety of brain disorders.

Donepezil (Aricept) for Mild Memory Loss

There are more and more people like Diane Pozniak who are taking donepezil (Aricept) for memory loss. Some, like Diane, have very mild symptoms that fall beneath most clinicians' scanning radar, while others have more clear-cut symptoms that can be called mild to moderate memory loss without dementia. After all, if donepezil is successful in improving memory in a condition like Alzheimer's that is horrendously difficult to treat, why shouldn't it work as well, or even better, for milder forms of memory loss? As Diane's story demonstrates, there is a place for donepezil in such a situation. In fact, recent studies suggest that it has a broad array of actions in improving memory: patients with multiple sclerosis show improved memory on donepezil compared to placebo, and patients taking antidepressants and similar medications (some with known anticholinergic effects) report a subjective improvement in memory on donepezil. (There was no objective memory testing or placebo control in that study, so view the results with caution.)

Before you run off to get a prescription of donepezil (Aricept) from your doctor, it is important for you to understand exactly how cholinergic medications work; this will give you a sound basis on which to make your decision to take or not to take Aricept.

Science in Evolution: The Cholinergic Story

In 1976, Peter Davies, who was examining autopsied brains of patients with Alzheimer's disease, reported the death of nerve cells that normally produced the neurotransmitter acetylcholine. Around the same time, David Drachman showed that administering scopolamine, which is an antagonist of acetylcholine, to normal people could produce memory impairment and other cognitive deficits that mimicked Alzheimer's disease. These discoveries began the race to develop an effective medication that could reverse the acetylcholine deficit seen in patients with Alzheimer's disease.

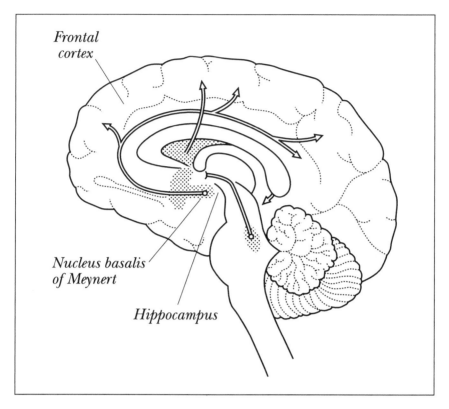

*Frontal
cortex*

*Nucleus basalis
of Meynert*

Hippocampus

Figure 3.   Cholinergic projections in the brain.

Nerve cells that release the neurotransmitter acetylcholine form the cholinergic system in the brain, which is divided into two parts: muscarinic (main focus of attention in memory) and nicotinic. The muscarinic projections are outlined in Figure 3, which represents a midline slice through the whole brain. Specific masses of nerve cells, or nuclei, in the deep part of the brain form the center of the muscarinic cholinergic system, and they use acetylcholine as their neurotransmitter. Degeneration of these cholinergic nerve cells deep in the brain leads to damage to the areas to which they project and are connected, namely, the hippocampus and frontal cortex. Naturally, memory loss is the result.

Role of Acetylcholine in Cognition
- Increase in acetylcholine leads to improved attention, mental arousal, and memory.

- From age forty to ninety, the nucleus basalis of Meynert gradually and progressively loses up to half its cholinergic nerve cells.
- This loss of cholinergic nerve cells causes a delay in the brain's ability to process information quickly and accurately, which is why aging leads to slower reactions as well as to mild memory loss.
- In Alzheimer's disease, the nucleus basalis is nearly wiped out within a few years after clinical onset of the illness, causing severe memory loss.

Cholinergic nerve cells release acetylcholine into a narrow cleft or space called the synapse. This acetylcholine molecule races across the synapse and latches onto a receptor in the next neuron, called the postsynaptic neuron. The postsynaptic receptor is specially configured for the acetylcholine molecule, the way a keyhole receives a key. Attachment to this receptor triggers a series of biochemical and physiologic events in the postsynaptic or receiving neuron, leading to a change in brain function that involves improved mental arousal and memory. Once acetylcholine completes its job, it is either sucked back by the nerve cell that released it, ready to fight another day, or it is broken down by the enzyme acetylcholinesterase in the synaptic cleft.

Different Ways to Boost Acetylcholine

Cholinesterase inhibitors are compounds that inhibit the action of this enzyme, acetylcholinesterase. Treatment with cholinesterase inhibitors indirectly raises the level of acetylcholine by preventing its breakdown, thereby leading to improved attention, mental arousal, learning, and memory. In fact, cholinesterase inhibitors have now reached the forefront of treatment in Alzheimer's disease, and memory loss more broadly.

If you step back for a moment and think about the issue, this indirect approach does seem a bit odd. Why not directly increase the amount of acetylcholine by pouring it directly into the synapse, or administer a substance (precursor) that is converted to acetylcholine in the brain? Well, these strategies have been tried with compounds like choline and lecithin.

Choline

Choline is directly converted into acetylcholine by combining with acetic acid, and you might think that choline should work quite well as a memory enhancer. Unfortunately, although animal studies show that choline heightens attention and helps to transfer information from short to long-term memory, the clinical data are inconsistent and unimpressive. Several placebo-controlled trials to treat Alzheimer's disease have met with failure. Similar efforts with choline have not worked in people with mild to moderate memory loss. To produce even the slightest effect, choline needs to be ingested in huge quantities of 3 to 12 grams daily. Another practical problem is that if you take this substance, you may exude a fishy smell, not a very appetizing prospect for bystanders, let alone your loved ones.

Lecithin

- Lecithin is an essential ingredient of living cells.
- It prevents cholesterol accumulation in arteries, and helps prevent liver degeneration.
- Phosphatidylcholine is the active element in lecithin that works against memory loss.
- Phosphatidylcholine is broken down to choline, which the body then uses to synthesize acetylcholine.
- Lecithin has a prolonged duration of action and needs to be taken only once or twice a day.

Like choline, in more than a dozen controlled studies of Alzheimer's patients, lecithin's effects have been very small and quite inconsistent. Similar results have emerged from the few placebo-controlled studies of lecithin to treat mild to moderate memory loss; there have been no studies to prevent age-related memory loss.

Your average daily diet contains approximately 1 gram of lecithin, but this is too little to have any promemory effects. You need to take a large amount—2 to 10 grams a day—to produce a very small, and debatable, improvement in memory. Lecithin can be purchased in health food stores. The amount of the vital component, phosphatidylcholine, varies from 25 to 55 percent in content in these products. The higher the proportion of phosphatidylcholine, the more likely lecithin may have a mild cognitive-enhancing effect.

The relative failure of choline and lecithin, medications that directly enhance cholinergic function, brings us back to the indirect strategy that led to the development and success of donepezil (Aricept): inhibition of the enzyme acetylcholinesterase. No one really understands exactly why, but this indirect route works much better than the direct approach. Among the cholinesterase inhibitors, physostigmine, acetyl-l-carnitine, tacrine, and donepezil are the most prominent.

Physostigmine

Studies with the cholinesterase inhibitor physostigmine in small numbers of Alzheimer's patients, some of which were conducted by my colleagues Drs. Yaakov Stern and Richard Mayeux, showed superior memory test performance compared to placebo. The size of the improvement was comparable to what would be shown years later with tacrine and donepezil, but physostigmine never succeeded in the same fashion for two main reasons: the very short duration of action meant that pills needed to be given five to six times daily, and it frequently caused nausea and other side effects. Given these difficulties, using physostigmine to prevent age-related memory loss was never even entertained as a concept. A long-acting physostigmine compound with single daily dosing was developed, but this did not prove to be very effective, and physostigmine is now consigned to the dust heap of history. I feel that this is unfortunate, because several of the Alzheimer's patients who participated in the clinical trials at our center did show some benefit.

Properties of Acetyl-l-carnitine (Alcar)

- Is found in muscle and helps get energy out of fat.
- Can repair damage in lymphocytes, a type of white blood cell that is essential for normal immune function.
- Boosts metabolism within nerve cells, and slows the loss of nerve growth factor that helps maintain the functioning of nerve cells in the hippocampus and frontal cortex. In fact, acetyl-l-carnitine raises the levels of nerve growth factor by 30 to 40 percent in the brains of rats.
- Prevents the loss of acetylcholinesterase, thereby indirectly enhancing cholinergic function.

While it remains unclear which of these many actions underlies acetyl-l-carnitine's promemory effects, I have chosen to discuss it under the cholinesterase inhibitor class of compounds.

Promising results emerged in small numbers of patients with Alzheimer's disease, but larger placebo-controlled trials met with failure. Other small-scale studies have shown an advantage for acetyl-l-carnitine over placebo in people with mild memory loss, but there are also several negative reports. Like other compounds in its class, there are no long-term studies to determine if it can prevent age-related memory loss.

The usual dose is 2 to 5 grams daily, and there are few side effects. You can obtain acetyl-l-carnitine in health food stores, and this is an example of how the same substance can surface as both a modern pharmaceutical compound and an alternative medication. In fact, as more and more research is conducted with various types of alternative medicines, the two fields will begin to converge and their boundaries may eventually disappear altogether.

The Rise and Fall of Tacrine (Cognex)

As the largely negative clinical trials with choline, lecithin, and acetyl-l-carnitine demonstrate, promemory effects in rats or mice are not easy to replicate in people. Improving cognition in the primitive rodent brain is a lot simpler than boosting it in the ultracomplex human brain.

As a matter of fact, by the mid 1980s, research with a variety of cholinergic compounds—lecithin, choline, phosphatidylcholine, acetyl-l-carnitine, and physostigmine—had run into a dead end, despite the investment of over a billion dollars by a number of drug companies in the United States, Europe, and Japan. Then came a report by William Koopmans Summers describing strong efficacy for a cholinesterase inhibitor named tetrahydroaminoacridine or tacrine (THA, Cognex) in seventeen patients with Alzheimer's disease. A tortuous road ensued for tacrine, with many ups and downs and the U.S. Congress getting involved in supporting research and development of this Warner Lambert drug. Eventually, the FDA approved it as a treatment for Alzheimer's disease, because high doses of the medication showed a significant, though small, advantage over placebo in cognitive performance.

But after tacrine was approved by the FDA, it fell by the wayside because of its liver toxicity. This risk was so high that after tacrine was approved for clinical use, none of the neurologists and psychiatrists in my group at Columbia University, including myself, were willing to prescribe the medication for our Alzheimer's patients, with rare exceptions. This situation changed dramatically with the development of the next FDA-approved cholinesterase inhibitor, donepezil (Aricept).

Donepezil (Aricept): A Rare Instance of Japan-U.S. Collaboration

Esai Pharmaceuticals, a Japanese company, did the basic research and initial clinical trials to develop donepezil (Aricept). Since they did not have a major presence in the United States, they cut a deal with Pfizer to conduct the required studies to obtain FDA approval and then to jointly market the medication in the United States and Europe. As one might expect, this Japan-U.S. collaboration has had its ups and downs, but both sides have learned a great deal in this process. Cross-border research and marketing will become increasingly important as drug development becomes more and more international, particularly if the byzantine regulations in different countries become more uniform.

Donepezil (Aricept) to Treat Alzheimer's Disease

In the double-blind study that provided the basis for obtaining FDA approval, outpatients with mild to moderate Alzheimer's disease were randomized to receive 10 mg donepezil daily (157 patients), 5 mg donepezil daily (154 patients), and placebo (162 patients). Both the 5 mg and 10 mg donepezil groups showed an average 3 to 8 percent advantage over placebo on cognitive performance and global clinical improvement. The peak effect occurred after six weeks on medication, and by six months the effect had begun to wear off. Nonetheless, throughout this period, patients on donepezil retained an advantage over patients who continued on placebo. In other words, the progress of Alzheimer's disease was not dramatically changed, but being on donepezil meant that the patient's worsening was delayed, unlike people on placebo, who deteriorated steadily over time.

From the original series of donepezil study participants, 133 Alzheimer's patients were followed for an average of two years. Donepezil treatment did not completely halt long-term decline, but it was associated with less deterioration than what was expected over time in these Alzheimer's patients.

Donepezil (Aricept):
The Prescription Choice for Mild Memory Loss

The success of donepezil in treating not only Alzheimer's disease but also some people with mild memory loss (like Diane Pozniak, described at the beginning of this chapter) has led the National Institute of Aging to launch a large-scale controlled study with both donepezil and vitamin E to find out how effective these medications are for people with mild to moderate memory loss. The results of that study are likely to have a major impact on the use of these two agents to treat mild memory loss, and as a preventive strategy for age-related memory loss.

Donepezil ranks at the top of my list of potentially useful prescription medications to prevent age-related memory loss, and to treat mild memory loss. Donepezil's cholinesterase inhibiting activity is similar to tacrine, but it has one great advantage: low toxicity. It has the added benefit of once-a-day dosing (5 or 10 mg). The main side effect is nausea or diarrhea, which affects a small number of people taking this medication. If your stomach can tolerate Aricept 5 mg daily, raising it to 10 mg daily should not present any problems. As with many new medications, Aricept is expensive ($3 to $6 daily).

Rivastigmine (Exelon)

Rivastigmine (Exelon) received FDA approval to treat Alzheimer's disease in May 2000, and it is a cholinesterase inhibitor that is very similar to donepezil (Aricept) in its clinical effects. Rivastigmine is given in doses of 3 to 12 mg daily but has to be taken twice (morning and evening), unlike the once-a-day dose for donepezil. Rivastigmine's common side effects include stomach upset, headache, and fatigue. More research is needed to find out if Exelon possesses any significant advantages over Aricept, but current information suggests few differences.

Other Cholinergic Compounds for Clinical Use

Currently, several pharmaceutical companies are trying to develop other cholinergic compounds to treat Alzheimer's disease (and mild memory loss), some of which are likely to be approved by the FDA during 2000–2001. Galantamine (Reminyl), which was provisionally approved by the FDA in late 2000, is very similar to donepezil (Aricept) and rivastigmine (Exelon) in its clinical effects. Galantamine is recommended in doses of 16 to 24 mg per day.

Nicotine Is a Cognitive Enhancer

There is another cholinergic system—nicotinic—in the brain that utilizes nicotine as its main neurotransmitter. Yes, this is the same nicotine that causes addiction to cigarettes! Nicotine stimulates the release of endorphins, which are the brain's natural morphinelike substances, and dopamine, which is involved in stimulating the reward-pleasure and arousal systems. The activating properties of nicotine, which make people more alert and aroused, may partly account for its addictive potential.

Nicotine receptors are deficient in the brains of patients with Alzheimer's disease. Initial studies using the nicotine skin patch in Alzheimer's patients were promising, but the latest studies have been negative. A broader question is whether nicotine can treat mild memory loss or prevent age-related memory loss. Early population-based studies suggested that smokers were less likely to develop Alzheimer's disease, but recent work has discounted this theory. Simultaneous administration of nicotinic and muscarinic compounds has never been attempted in any clinical trial, largely because of the fear of increased cholinergic toxicity. At this stage, the data on nicotine are insufficient for me to recommend it as a therapeutic or preventive strategy against memory loss.

Rational Choices

Enhancing cholinergic transmission using cholinergic compounds may be one of the most effective ways of treating, and possibly preventing, memory loss. Donepezil (Aricept) heads my recommended list, but high cost and the fact that it is a prescription medication are significant limitations. Exelon and Reminyl are alternatives to Aricept, but they are also expensive prescription medications. If you would like to try other options, particularly if you prefer natural substances that you can obtain in health food stores, you can consider acetyl-l-carnitine or lecithin. But I'd like you to remember that the data on these other medications are not as convincing as they are for Aricept (or Exelon or Reminyl). Regardless of which agent you choose, the standard approach is to start at the lowest dose and increase it gradually until you reach the maximum dose that you can tolerate without side effects. Do not take more than one of these medications simultaneously, because the risk of toxicity increases.

CHAPTER 18

Medications That Stimulate Brain Function

P HOSPHATIDYLSERINE, HYDERGINE, and nootropics act via brain mechanisms other than acetylcholine.

Phosphatidylserine (PS) for Age-Related Memory Loss

Phosphatidylserine is a naturally occurring substance that is chemically similar to phosphatidylcholine, which is the active promemory ingredient in lecithin. But what is the basis for its use, and where does it fit into your memory program?

Physiologic Actions of Phosphatidylserine
- Phosphatidylserine is present in the membrane that surrounds each cell, and it can alter the fluidity and functional state of these cell membranes. Stabilizing cell membranes may shield the nerve cell from injury and death.
- Phosphatidylserine indirectly increases the production and release of several neurotransmitters, including epinephrine, norepinephrine, serotonin, and dopamine. These neurotransmitters, especially norepinephrine and dopamine, are known to improve attention, concentration, and alertness.
- In aged mice, phosphatidylserine prevents, and partly reverses, age-related neurochemical changes. Mice receiving this com-

pound do not show the expected age-related decline in the ability to learn new information, such as figuring out how to traverse a maze.

Phosphatidylserine is a lipid, or fatty, substance and hence it crosses smoothly into the brain, unlike most water-soluble medications. This fat solubility makes it easy to navigate the blood-brain barrier, which is a natural boundary in capillaries or small blood vessels that prevents many substances in the bloodstream from entering the brain. After radioactively labeled phosphatidylserine is taken by mouth, it can be detected in the brain with high concentrations in the hippocampus and frontal cortex, areas responsible for memory.

Clinical Studies

Italian researchers evaluated phosphatidylserine in small-scale uncontrolled clinical trials, each in approximately thirty volunteer subjects who had minimal memory deficits. Phosphatidylserine showed memory-enhancing properties in these subjects. Later, several placebo-controlled trials were conducted, some by European researchers and a few by Dr. Thomas Crook, an American psychologist who has worked closely with the pharmaceutical companies in trying to find a treatment for "age-associated memory impairment." This narrow diagnostic category is defined by poor performance on a few neuropsychological tests, and represents only part of the population with age-related memory loss. In several studies of people with age-associated memory impairment, phosphatidylserine was superior to placebo on specific neuropsychological measures. If you tend to forget names, take heart: phosphatidylserine has been shown to be helpful for that very symptom. In these studies, the consistency, more than the size, of the cognitive improvement was impressive. Hence I place phosphatidylserine near the top of my list of medications that you can take for age-related memory loss, and to prevent the onset of age-related memory loss.

A Few Words of Caution

A few words of caution before you jump headfirst onto the phosphatidylserine bandwagon: nearly all studies so far have involved fewer than fifty people, meaning that fewer than twenty-five people received phosphatidylserine and fewer than twenty-five people received placebo. Also, the duration of these clinical trials was usually six to twelve weeks. We don't know if these people would have maintained cognitive improvement on phosphatidylserine over a period of several months to years, but this is quite possible.

Phosphatidylserine Products and Content

The amount of phosphatidylserine available in your diet, primarily through fish, soy beans, and green vegetables, is too little to have a significant promemory effect. The health food product derived from cow brains has given way to soy-based phosphatidylserine (mad cow disease was not responsible for this change), which should be of some comfort to those of you who are vegetarians. The content of phosphatidylserine varies among health food products. The label "Leci-PS" indicates that the product's contents have been tested by a standard laboratory to ensure that it contains adequate amounts of phosphatidylserine, as claimed by the manufacturer of that particular brand. "Brain gum," which contains phosphatidylserine, has gained popularity during the last few years.

Phosphatidylserine: Dosage and Side Effects

Phosphatidylserine (PS) 300 mg daily for six to eight weeks should be followed by 100 mg daily for maintenance therapy, based on the notion that a smaller dose is sufficient after the neuronal cell membranes have been saturated with phosphatidylserine. Astonishingly, the research studies indicate virtually no side effects. This makes the physician in me slightly nervous, because the medication without any side effects has yet to be invented. In particular, the possible side effects of long-term daily intake have not been properly assessed. If phosphatidylserine is used by tens of thousands of people, it is likely that we will hear more about its side effects, especially side effects that occur in only a small subgroup of vulnerable individuals.

Given the fair amount of information available on the use of PS to treat mild memory loss, it is somewhat surprising that it has not caught the public's attention. A large proportion of patients with mild memory loss who come to our Memory Disorders Center take vitamin E or ginkgo biloba, but hardly anyone takes PS. One reason may be that there has been no large-scale clinical trial in Alzheimer's disease, which is necessary for any compound to reach the headlines as a treatment for memory loss. But the fact that most phosphatidylserine studies were conducted in people who had mild memory loss, and not clinical disorders like Alzheimer's disease, is an added plus for your purposes.

Hydergine: The First FDA-Approved Antidementia Medication

Hydergine is derived from ergot alkaloids (present in rye fungus) that are also used in antimigraine medications. The drug company Sandoz (now part of Novartis) began to study hydergine after it learned that ergot alkaloids were used by nontraditional practitioners to lower a pregnant mother's blood pressure during childbirth. Sandoz's goal was to use hydergine to lower blood pressure and the risk of stroke; this didn't pan out, but they did manage to get it approved as a treatment for dementia.

From the 1980s into the early 1990s, I saw a large number of patients suffering from dementia who took hydergine. General practitioners or internists usually prescribed it to these patients. On occasion, I myself prescribed hydergine to patients with dementia when, out of desperation, family members insisted that I prescribe something, anything, even if there wasn't any solid evidence supporting the medication's use.

At that time, hydergine was the only medication approved in the United States for the treatment of dementia. If the data on this compound were presented to today's hypervigilant FDA, it probably would not win approval as a memory-enhancing medication. In the patients with dementia who took hydergine, I observed the following:

- no change in memory
- a rare patient or two who became more alert with increased mental arousal
- no obvious side effects at the standard doses recommended in the *Physicians' Desk Reference* (*PDR*)

In other words, I thought of it as similar to placebo, but in the absence of other available options, it wasn't such a bad choice. My approach in prescribing such a medication was to make the patient and family members fully aware that the chances of significant improvement were extremely low, but that it might be worth a shot given the lack of other available options.

Properties of Hydergine

1. Increases blood flow and glucose utilization in the brain.
2. Indirectly helps decrease free-radical formation.
3. Stimulates the production of the neurotransmitters norepinephrine and dopamine, which help to maintain attention and alertness (mental arousal, vigilance). These actions may

account for hydergine's activating and mild mood-elevating effects, which occur in some people.

The Bottom Line on Hydergine

As you may have gathered, I am not a great fan of hydergine, and neither are most physicians these days. I think of it as a mildly activating agent in some cases, without any measurable effect on memory. The advent of vitamin E, ginkgo biloba, cholinesterase inhibitors, phosphatidylserine, and several other promemory agents has pushed hydergine far into the background. Most physicians have stopped prescribing hydergine because there are so many other treatment options. If you or someone close to you is on hydergine, note that the standard U.S. prescription dose is 3 mg per day, but in Europe doses of 9 to 12 mg per day are often prescribed without any apparent problems. In a few countries like Mexico, you can get hydergine over-the-counter. Since it is off patent, you can now get cheaper generic products even in the United States. The main advantage is that there are very few side effects with this medication. Nausea, stomach upset, and headache can rarely occur, but these symptoms tend to be mild.

Nootropics: Drugs Meant to Make You Smarter

Nootropics, called "smart drugs" by some aficionados, refer to a wide range of potential memory-enhancing medications. Over time, the term has become restricted to describe a relatively narrow class of medications. Nootropics were developed with the idea that they would work not only for people with memory disorders but would also improve cognitive performance in normal individuals. The hope was that somehow these medications would help nerve cells sprout and form connections with other nerve cells, but there are no sound experimental data to back this idea.

Piracetam, oxiracetam, aniracetam, and pramiracetam (all derived from pyrrolidone) are the most widely used nootropic compounds.

Actions of Piracetam and Related Nootropics
- In animal studies, they increase glucose metabolism in nerve cells.
- In other animal studies, piracetam increased the number of acetylcholine receptors and the amount of acetylcholine released into synapses.
- In the laboratory, nootropics can boost memory in animals and reverse memory loss induced by toxic drugs.

- Piracetam may improve communication between the right and left halves of the brain. Since this informational transfer and integration may be linked to creativity, many artists and writers in Europe take it for this purpose.
- Piracetam has a very small effect in enhancing cognitive performance in normal elderly people and in children with learning disabilities. It may improve attention span and the integration of information.
- Nootropics are claimed to minimize damage from stroke; data are minimal.

Nootropics to Treat Dementia

Efforts to use piracetam by itself to treat Alzheimer's disease have met with failure. In a handful of Alzheimer's patients, combining piracetam with choline for a week led to some improvement. Piracetam's ability to increase cholinergic transmission suggests that combining it with cholinesterase inhibitors like donepezil may be a good idea, but this approach has not been tested in long-term clinical trials. In a small study, pramiracetam seemed to work against memory loss in patients who previously suffered head injuries. Unfortunately, most nootropic research has been fairly shoddy and often misused to make fairly tall claims about their clinical utility.

The main advantage of all the nootropics is that they are relatively harmless, with few to no side effects. Doses of pramiracetam, for example, can range from 12.5 mg all the way to 400 mg daily, and most patients do not experience side effects even at the highest dose.

Piracetam, the main nootropic medication, has been marketed since 1972, and is available in more than eighty countries, including many in Europe, but not in the United States. Inconsistent results have failed to convince the FDA to give its stamp of approval to any nootropic as a treatment for dementia or other memory disorders.

Nootropics Don't Help Age-Associated Memory Impairment

Tom Crook conducted a number of studies with nootropics in subjects with age-associated memory impairment. After investing a great deal of time, energy, and pharmaceutical industry money, he concluded that nootropics like piracetam and pramiracetam cannot be recommended as a treatment for mild memory loss during the aging process. I agree and am not including this class of compounds in my recommended list of promemory medications.

CHAPTER 19

Estrogen

Cynthia's Story

Cynthia Holmes, an elderly African-American woman, began with the statement that she was not sure if she was coming to the right place. Her sister thought she was getting depressed and her friends told her she was not as mentally sharp as she used to be, but Cynthia herself felt that her problems were too minor to merit seeing a doctor. The ravages of osteoarthritis had reduced her height from six feet to five feet nine inches, and she shuffled into my office looking as if a strong wind was behind her back, bending her over. Her face was heavily lined with wrinkles, and she displayed a listless, apathetic look. I guessed that she was around eighty years old, but in fact she was only sixty-four. She said she was forgetting names more often, found it difficult to keep track of her checks and monthly bills, and tended to forget the sequence of cards during games that she occasionally played with friends. She also reported low energy and fatigue, and a loss of interest in crocheting and other hobbies that she used to enjoy. She had retired at the age of sixty from a clerical job, and since that time she had developed a somewhat negative, pessimistic outlook on life. She did not have any difficulty in sleeping, there was no change in her appetite, and her interest in sex was lower than what it used to be, a change that she attributed to the loss of her husband from a stroke eight years earlier.

    She did not feel that she had significant memory loss or depression because, as she put it, "You know, I think it's normal to lose your memory a little, to feel a bit low about getting old. My body doesn't function the way it should. Many in my family have died, and some of my friends have passed away too. At my age, I don't see how things are going to get better for me."

She had come to our Memory Disorders Center at the insistence of her sister Myra, who had become worried about the changes that she had observed. When Myra walked into the office a few minutes later, the contrast between the two women was so striking that I momentarily wondered if the two were even related. Myra was well built, bouncy on her feet, and had a jovial, lively manner that lit up her face and was quite endearing.

"Your older sister was just telling me that she is no longer as interested in her hobbies," I said.

Myra looked at her sister Cynthia, turned toward me with a puzzled expression, and then suddenly laughed. "You kiddin' me? She's not older. Cynthia, my little sister? She's six years younger than I am!"

I simply couldn't believe it. I had guessed that Myra was fifty, not seventy years old. And with my earlier impression of Cynthia being eighty rather than sixty-four, the contrast between the two sisters was even more striking to me. So I asked Myra about her own health habits. She went through the usual litany: a sound diet, regular exercise, no smoking, low alcohol intake, and a mellow, low-stress approach to life. Finally, she revealed that she was taking Premarin, a standard estrogen-replacement therapy for postmenopausal women.

I turned to ask her sister Cynthia if she had thought of taking estrogen herself.

"My aunt died of breast cancer, so I won't take the risk," she replied.

Myra explained that she had no problems on estrogen and that she had regular, frequent checkups with her gynecologist, including regular mammograms and pelvic exams. But Cynthia remained adamant that because there was a risk of cancer, she would not take estrogen.

Keeping this information in the front of my mind, I completed the diagnostic workup for Cynthia's memory loss, and possible depression. There were no abnormalities on neurological examination or any laboratory test, including MRI scan of the brain. Her neuropsychological testing showed only minimal deficits, which may have been due to mild depression. A twelve-week treatment course with the antidepressant medication paroxetine led to only slight improvement in her symptoms. Other antidepressant medications met the same fate. She refused to consider psychotherapy. She also did not want to try any memory-enhancing exercises or related techniques, so I asked her to start taking vitamin E 800 IUs daily. Adding the cholinesterase inhibitor donepezil (Aricept) had no significant impact on her memory. Cynthia's general health habits (sound diet, regular walks, no alcohol) were very good, so there wasn't much room for improvement there.

Over the next two years, Cynthia did not change very much. Occasional memory lapses persisted, but without any worsening over time. Her neuropsychological testing showed no significant changes during this period. My attempts to get her to reconsider estrogen therapy, or at least to discuss it with her gynecologist, were met with stony refusal. Her older sister Myra, who accompanied Cynthia for some of her clinic visits, continued on her youthful, estrogen-filled way without any major health problems.

The main female sex hormone, estrogen, is produced by the ovaries. As Cynthia and Myra illustrate, its actions extend far beyond reproduction and sexual behavior. For Myra, estrogen prevented not only memory decline but also the ravages of the aging process itself.

Effects of Estrogen
- Estrogen helps to prevent a common malady of old age: osteoarthritis, in which bone decay leads to generalized weakness, altered gait, and a stooped posture.
- Postmenopausal women who take estrogen may actually increase their life span.
- Estrogen's effects in the brain are less well recognized, but a lack of this hormone can give rise to memory loss.

Genetic Factors Influence Treatment Response

In all branches of medicine, there is a general rule that genetic factors play an important role in predicting treatment response. If one family member responds to a treatment, the other family member will likely respond to the same treatment. I am convinced that estrogen could have accomplished for Cynthia what it had achieved for Myra, and that its effects on both mild depression and memory loss would have been far greater than the standard antidepressant and antimemory-loss medications that she received. My guess is that her primary problem was estrogen deficiency (blood estrogen levels are not very useful and don't tell us how well estrogen is being utilized in the brain), which is why the other treatments did not work as well as they usually do.

Estrogen in Long-Term Prevention of Memory Loss

Clinical anecdotes and observations about the power of estrogen have been supported by the results from systematic studies, especially of elderly women living at home. In a report from the Baltimore Longitudinal Study on Normal Aging, 472 menopausal and postmenopausal women were followed for sixteen years. Women on estrogen-replacement therapy were 50 percent less likely to develop dementia. Other studies of women living in the community have also shown that estrogen provides a protective effect against dementia. Most of these studies suggest a twofold to fourfold protective effect, meaning that if you are sixty years old and your risk of getting dementia in the next ten years is 12 percent, this risk will drop to 3 to 6 percent if you are taking estrogen. No one is suggesting that estrogen will cure Alzheimer's, but rather that the procognition properties of estrogen will delay the onset of the disease by several years. The results of several studies indicate that the longer you take estrogen, and the higher the dose, the greater the protective effect against this dreaded disease.

Estrogen Therapy for Memory Loss

In a study that used the cholinergic medication tacrine (Cognex) to treat Alzheimer's disease, an incidental result was that women who also took estrogen were the patients most likely to improve cognitively with tacrine. This intriguing result suggests that estrogen may be particularly effective when used in combination with other medications.

Recent studies suggest that estrogen by itself is not an effective treatment for Alzheimer's disease. However, other studies show that estrogen may slightly enhance memory performance in postmenopausal women who do not suffer from memory loss. My view is that estrogen may be particularly effective in women who have symptoms of both depression and cognitive impairment. This dovetails perfectly into the differences that I observed between the two sisters, with Cynthia suffering from mild depression and mild memory loss while Myra had neither syndrome and took estrogen.

Recently, several large-scale studies, including the Women's Health Initiative under the auspices of the NIH, have been launched to evaluate the direct effect of estrogen in preventing and treating mild memory loss. This massive investment means that it is likely that our knowledge about the effects of estrogen on memory will leapfrog over all the other promemory medications in the coming years.

How about a Male Estrogen?

How about a male estrogen to prevent not only memory loss but also heart attacks and strokes that are more common in men than in women? There is work afoot to try to develop compounds that retain many of the properties of estrogen without producing its feminizing effects such as changes in breast size and other physical features. The antiosteoporosis medication raloxifene (Evista), which some have informally labeled as estrogen-light, has fewer feminizing properties than regular estrogen, but it is still not suitable for use by men. A recent study in women showed that Evista was much less likely to lead to breast cancer than estrogen, and this compound may be worth testing in women with mild memory loss.

The irony about estrogen is that it is a steroid, as is the male hormone, testosterone. Corticosteroids are thought to damage hippocampal cells, but sex hormone steroids may actually protect the same cells. Testosterone therapy in men has not been studied as much as estrogen in women for a couple of reasons: a high risk of prostate cancer, and the need to give testosterone by injection rather than orally. Since more and more researchers are taking an interest in sex hormones and related compounds, male sex hormone therapy to prevent memory loss, and perhaps depression, may make its debut in the future.

How Estrogen Works in the Brain

Estrogen has the following effects that individually or together may be responsible for its promemory actions:

1. Promotes the growth and survival of cholinergic nerve cells in the brain, probably by stimulating a substance called nerve growth factor.

2. May reduce destructive amyloid formation that occurs to a small extent during normal aging and to a precipitous degree in Alzheimer's disease.
3. May diminish the inflammatory response in the brain. Abnormal immune reactions are believed to underlie many brain disorders and may contribute to age-related memory loss.
4. Helps to maintain synapses, which are the small gaps between nerve cells bridged by chemical neurotransmitters. This action may prolong the integrity and life of synapses that normally decay during the aging process.
5. Has moderate antioxidant properties.
6. Raising estrogen levels in mice improves performance on memory tasks such as remembering how to traverse a maze.

Types and Dosage of Estrogen

There are different types of estrogen in the blood and in the brain—estriol and estradiol, for example—but they are all fairly similar in their actions. For postmenopausal women, estrogen ranks high on my list of medications to prevent age-related memory loss, and as a potential treatment for mild memory loss. If you have had a hysterectomy, the simplest therapeutic approach is to take conjugated estrogen, which is marketed as Premarin. The standard Premarin dose is a single tablet of 0.625 mg daily. If you have not had a hysterectomy, it is necessary to add progesterone, which is the other main female hormone. Combining the two reduces the risk of cancer of the uterus. You can achieve this by taking a single daily tablet of an estrogen-progesterone combination that contains 0.625 mg Premarin and 2.5 mg medroxyprogesterone acetate. There are over a dozen brands of estrogen-progesterone combinations on the market, but they are all about the same. They are all prescription medications, and you need to work out the exact doses, as well as the timing sequence of estrogen and progesterone therapy, with your doctor (internist or gynecologist).

Risks of Estrogen Therapy

Estrogen therapy stimulates estrogen-responsive cells in the breast and uterus, and hence slightly raises the risk of both breast and uterine cancer. A family history of breast or uterine cancer is a cautionary sign, but by itself it does not mean you shouldn't take estrogen. Cynthia was unwilling to take the risk because her aunt had suffered from breast cancer. Her sister Myra did take the risk and benefited greatly from estrogen replacement therapy. During the last couple of decades, improved technology in early breast cancer detection has tilted the balance in favor of estrogen therapy, which is why I recommended it for Cynthia.

There is a small risk of clotting with inflammation of the veins—thrombophlebitis—which most commonly affects the leg veins. In rare cases, this can affect the larger leg veins and cause deep vein thrombosis, which is a potentially dangerous complication because the thrombus or blood clot can enter the veins and lodge in the blood vessels that supply the lungs. If you have a history of this type of complication either while taking birth control pills or during pregnancy, do not take estrogen.

Other side effects include breast discomfort and resumption of uterine bleeding in postmenopausal women who have not had a hysterectomy, though this depends on the timing sequence of the estrogen-progesterone combination. If you take estrogen, you will need to be monitored by a physician, preferably a gynecologist, for side effects and complications using regular mammograms, ultrasound if necessary, pap smears, and pelvic/radiologic examinations.

CHAPTER 20

Brain Inflammation

INFLAMMATION IS THE BODY'S REACTION to infection or injury, causing symptoms of pain, redness, swelling, and warmth. Medications like acetylsalicylic acid (aspirin) suppress the inflammatory response. To better understand how anti-inflammatory compounds can help prevent memory loss, you need to have some basic knowledge about the workings of the immune system, which is responsible for the process of inflammation.

The Immune System

There are two main types of immunity: cell-mediated and humoral. Cell-mediated immunity relies on specialized cells in the body to isolate, surround, and destroy the offender. The white blood cells are the generals in charge of this defense department. They roam through the bloodstream, attacking and destroying all infiltrators and spies: bacteria and viruses, toxins and allergens. If too many white blood cells get bogged down dealing with invaders, extra reinforcements pour out of the bone marrow into the blood to fight the battle.

The second type of immunity, called humoral, is the immune system's antibody response to a foreign substance (antigen). The antibody is a protein that forms a perfect physical and chemical fit to the antigen molecule, and thus neutralizes it. This antibody response can go haywire and produce allergies, hay fever, and asthma. The body has the capacity to produce new antibodies, or antidotes, to thousands of different compounds or antigens, like a chemical factory that can

181

change the substance it produces at will. Occasionally, a hyperactive immune system can mistakenly attack the body's own tissues, as happens in rheumatoid arthritis and lupus. On the flip side, a weak immune system that does not destroy wayward cancerous cells can lead to malignant tumor formation, as occurs in AIDS.

Inflammation in the Alzheimer's Brain

Within the brain, the immune system interacts closely with nerve cells in several regions and is triggered in a variety of ways. The complement pathway (a sequence of enzymes/proteins) plays an important role in the immune response, and an overactive complement response can damage different areas of the brain. In patients with Alzheimer's disease, complement activation can trigger the formation of amyloid protein that collects in clumps to make up the pathologic amyloid plaques. Researchers are now studying anti-inflammatory agents that can block or inactivate complement in the treatment of not only Alzheimer's disease, but also mild to moderate memory loss during the aging process.

Types of Anti-inflammatory Agents

Anti-inflammatory medications are of two types: steroidal and nonsteroidal. It may seem odd that steroids, which in high concentrations can damage the hippocampus, can be therapeutic for patients with dementia. However, the fact that inflammation does occur in the brains of these patients suggests that steroids, which have extremely powerful anti-inflammatory properties, may indeed be effective treatments. Drs. Paul Aisen and Ken Davis at the Mount Sinai Medical Center in New York certainly think so, and they recently completed a placebo-controlled clinical trial using prednisone, a synthetic steroid, in Alzheimer's disease. However, the trial results were negative: prednisone showed no advantage over placebo in these patients.

The other approach is to use nonsteroidal anti-inflammatory medications (NSAIDs) like acetylsalicylic acid (aspirin), indomethacin (Indocin), or ibuprofen (Motrin). Acetaminophen (Tylenol) has weak anti-inflammatory properties compared to aspirin, even though it has similar pain-killing strength.

Lessons from Arthritis

In rheumatoid arthritis, the kind that causes swelling and deformity of the fingers and toes, as well as the hands and feet, the body's immune system mistakenly identifies joint tissue parts as alien and attacks them with a vengeance. Since many people who suffer from this disease regularly have to take high doses of anti-inflammatory medications, the question arises: do these people have a lower prevalence of dementia, especially Alzheimer's disease, compared to the rest of the population?

Patrick McGeer and his colleagues at the University of British Columbia in Canada conducted a comprehensive review of seventeen studies conducted in nine countries to evaluate the associations between the use of anti-inflammatory medications and Alzheimer's disease. They concluded that the use of either NSAIDs or steroids cuts the risk of having Alzheimer's disease by approximately half. This finding held up whichever way the data were analyzed: looking at the presence of rheumatoid arthritis alone, the use of either NSAIDs or steroids, or a combination of these treatments. Some of these effects of nonsteroidal medications in Alzheimer's disease and stroke may also apply to treatment and prevention of mild memory loss.

Taking Anti-inflammatory Agents for Memory Loss

In a survey of people living at home, John Breitner of Duke University discovered that elderly people who were taking anti-inflammatory agents like aspirin and ibuprofen were less likely to get dementia than the rest of the population. Breitner has continued this work after moving to Johns Hopkins, and has found a protective effect for NSAIDs against dementia in a large study of twins. Other reports from Johns Hopkins showed that Alzheimer's patients who took NSAIDs performed better on neuropsychological tests. Approaching the same problem from a different angle, Japanese researchers demonstrated that the use of dapsone, which is an antileprosy agent with anti-inflammatory properties, was associated with a significantly lower risk of developing Alzheimer's disease.

Placebo-controlled trials using both over-the-counter and prescription anti-inflammatory medications have involved very few subjects, but the results are quite intriguing. J. Rogers and colleagues at the Sun Health Research Institute in Arizona conducted a six-month study using the NSAID indomethacin (Indocin) and placebo in twenty-eight patients with Alzheimer's disease. Patients on indomethacin showed an average 1.3 percent improvement in cognitive performance compared to an 8.4 percent worsening in the placebo group, a significant difference.

The Pros and Cons of Aspirin

Aspirin remains the top choice among anti-inflammatory agents, because it has two more promemory actions: antioxidant activity by trapping hydroxyl radicals, and anticlotting property that helps prevent stroke.

Personal experience makes me a trifle wary of recommending aspirin for everyone. A few years ago, after my mother had a balloon angioplasty for unstable angina, her cardiologist started her on a single tablet of aspirin 325 mg daily. A few days later, she noticed blood in the stools. I suggested to her cardiologist that the aspirin be stopped. Barely five days had elapsed since the angioplasty, so he was loath to discontinue the aspirin, because he wanted to prevent recurrence of blood clots in the coronary arteries that supply the heart. Eventually, after considerable coaxing from me, he agreed to reduce my mother's dose to a baby aspirin (81 mg) daily. A couple of days later, she had further, massive lower gastrointestinal bleeding, and I rushed her to the emergency room. It was touch and go for a while, and she required six pints of blood in the intensive care unit before she was stabilized. After an endoscopic examination, the consultant gastroenterologist found evidence of bleeding and educated me about the fact that aspirin can cause bleeding from not only the stomach but also lower down in the intestines. This explained why my mother had both upper and lower gastrointestinal bleeding that was so severe it had dropped her hemoglobin to one-third the normal concentration in the blood. She was then switched to ticlopidine (Ticlid) and later to clopidogrel (Plavix), which have anticoagulant properties similar to aspirin. Obviously, she has not been within a hundred feet of an aspirin tablet since that time.

While this degree of exquisite sensitivity to aspirin is quite rare, I hope this makes you realize that even aspirin is not an entirely harmless medication. In fact, if aspirin were presented today to the FDA as a new drug, it might not be approved because of its high toxicity.

COX-II Inhibitors and the Future

If anti-inflammatory agents can prevent or slow down the progression of Alzheimer's disease, then could they also work against milder forms of memory loss? Merck, the pharmaceutical company that manufactures rofecoxib (Vioxx), one of the new Cyclo-oxygenase (COX)-II inhibitors that has been approved by the FDA to treat arthritis, has started a large-scale placebo-controlled clinical trial to evaluate the new medication's effects in treating people with mild cognitive impairment. Similarly, Searle, which makes another COX-II inhibitor called celecoxib (Celebrex), is completing a similar trial in people with mild cognitive impairment.

These COX-II inhibitors hold some promise as promemory agents. Other drug companies are likely to develop similar compounds. These new medications are as powerful as older NSAIDs, and because they preferentially enter the brain more than the rest of the body, they seem to be less likely to cause the side effects of stomach irritation, ulcers, and bleeding.

Therapeutic Guidelines for Anti-inflammatory Medications

For anti-inflammatory agents, a few broad guidelines are in order. Although steroids like prednisone have the strongest anti-inflammatory properties, these are fairly toxic compounds that are quite tricky to use. In addition, the negative results in the recent Alzheimer's study have convinced me to exclude steroids from the Memory Program.

Among the NSAIDs, the antioxidant and anticoagulant properties of aspirin give it a slight edge over the other available compounds. If you have risk factors for stroke or heart attack—for example, a strong family history or a high cholesterol blood level—an aspirin a day is a good idea. It may also protect against memory loss, given its antistroke and anti-inflammatory properties. Other NSAIDs like ibuprofen (Motrin) or indomethacin (Indocin) also irritate the stomach lining, though to a lesser extent than aspirin (enteric-coated or buffered aspirin helps but does not always solve the problem). The other NSAIDs do not share aspirin's anticoagulant properties that help reduce the risk of stroke and heart attacks.

Our best hope for the use of anti-inflammatory agents to prevent memory loss lies with the new COX-II inhibitors. We should know about the results of the Merck and Searle trials to treat mild to moderate memory loss within the next couple of years, and if they are positive, these medications could become the linchpin of a therapeutic strategy against memory loss due to the aging process. The relative lack of side effects will allow most people to take these medications without difficulty. Stay tuned for the results of the COX-II inhibitor trials in people with mild to moderate memory loss.

PART FIVE

Putting It All Together

CHAPTER 21

Your Comprehensive Memory Program

One must have a good memory to be able to keep the
promises one makes.
—F. W. NIETZSCHE

Become familiar with all aspects of the Memory Program
before you decide which of these components you wish to employ in
your own life. If you have reached this far in the book, you know that
the Memory Program must be tailored to the individual.

Much of the material in this chapter follows directly from what
I covered in earlier chapters. To reiterate, there is no magic memory pill, no silver bullet. To help preserve and even improve your
memory, a comprehensive, multifaceted program is the right solution.

The Memory Program is intended to help two categories of
people:

1. Those who currently have a normal memory and wish to preserve their memory during the aging process. If you're in
your forties or fifties, you probably fall into this category.
2. Those with mild memory loss who would like to reverse the
process or at least prevent further decline. If you're in your
sixties to eighties, you may fall into this category. However,

189

you can develop mild memory loss in your forties or fifties, especially if you have a specific, usually reversible, cause of memory loss such as depression, alcohol abuse, medication toxicity, or hypothyroidism.

If You've Developed Mild Memory Loss, What Does It Mean?

- If you are in your forties to fifties, you are likely to have an identifiable, reversible cause of memory loss.
- If you are in your sixties to eighties, memory loss due to either the aging process or dementia is much more common.
- If there is a relatively rapid onset (weeks to months) of symptoms, a potentially reversible cause of memory loss is likely.
- A fluctuating course of symptoms, with periods of clear memory and cognition intervening between episodes of confusion or memory loss, is more likely to be due to an identifiable, reversible cause.
- A gradual dwindling in memory over many years, even decades, is typical of memory loss due to the aging process.
- A steady decline, with mild symptoms progressing to severe symptoms of memory loss within a few years, suggests Alzheimer's disease.

Early benign signs of memory loss due to the aging process include forgetting names, forgetting a few items on a shopping list, misplacing keys, or not recognizing someone you met a long time ago. Signs of severe memory loss include getting lost in a familiar place, losing your way when driving a familiar route, forgetting important appointments repeatedly, forgetting to turn off the stove on many occasions, repeating the same questions over and over again, coworkers' pointing out that mistakes are increasing, and not knowing the date or time on several occasions.

If you have signs of severe memory loss, you need to see a doctor (neurologist or psychiatrist or primary care physician, preferably with a neuropsychologist's input). For those of you with mild memory loss, or if you have a sound memory but wish to prevent future memory loss, it's time to get into the nitty-gritty of the Memory Program.

The Memory Program

This comprehensive Memory Program has three major steps, each involving several components:

Step 1. Identifying and treating specific, reversible causes of memory loss;

Step 2. General measures to protect against memory loss that include a healthy diet, physical exercise, and memory training;

Step 3. Medication strategies to maintain and improve your memory.

I will first describe the Memory Program in its entirety, and then individualize the program by focusing on subcategories of people, based on whether you have a sound memory or mild memory loss, as well as by gender and age group.

Step 1: Identify Reversible Causes of Memory Loss

I have started with reversible causes of memory loss for a very important reason. If you fall within the category of people with mild memory loss, identifying and treating these reversible causes, where a cure is often possible, should be your first step. A large minority of people with mild memory loss suffer from reversible causes, and it is absolutely essential to fix these causes first.

The following table outlines the most common reversible causes of memory loss, and describes typical symptoms and the main treatment approaches for the specific disorder. To avoid clutter, less common causes like drug abuse and infections are not listed in the table. The symptoms of many of these reversible causes are not restricted to memory loss but also include general cognitive and intellectual decline.

If you suffer from mild memory loss and think you may be suffering from a potentially reversible cause:

1. Carefully read the relevant chapter earlier in this book and institute the recommended measures.
2. If you're not sure about whether you have a reversible cause, go see your doctor. Diagnosis and treatment of some reversible causes require physician consultation.

Reversible Causes and Age-Related Memory Loss: The Domino Effect

Returning to an earlier point, some people develop mild memory loss for the first time in their sixties and seventies. Many of these people

Common Reversible Causes of Memory Loss

Reversible Cause	Typical Symptoms	Diagnosis and Treatment
Stress	Easily distractible, forgetful Sense of inability to cope Flying off the handle frequently Excessive anxiety, palpitations Unable to enjoy vacations	Prune overload: do it constantly Focus on small not just big stressors Avoid conflict over trivial matters Regular bedtime hours, don't overeat Avoid late evening alcohol, caffeine Meditation, yoga, relaxation
Depression	Feeling low, down in the dumps Seeing the negative side of things Poor memory, unable to concentrate Loss of interest in hobbies, activities Insomnia, loss of appetite, low libido Daily tasks seem overwhelming Family history of depression	Maintain active social life Strengthen relationships Resolve outstanding conflicts If others say you look depressed, take the comment seriously and act on it Persistent, severe symptoms, seek help: psychotherapy, medications
Alcohol abuse	Drinking a little extra every day Hiding the truth about alcohol intake Critical comments from family, friends Gaps in memory for recent events	Reduce or eliminate alcohol intake Help from family, friends Alcoholics Anonymous Detoxification, specialized programs Vitamin B1 (thiamine)
Medication toxicity	Taking memory-toxic medications Poor attention, memory or confusion after starting a new medicine or dose increase of an existing medicine Change in sleep-wake cycle	Eliminate offending medication or reduce its dose Consult with your doctor regarding prescription medications
Thyroid deficiency	Memory loss, depression, lethargy Physical and mental slowness, weight gain, constipation, cold intolerance	Physician consultation Blood tests to confirm the diagnosis Thyroid hormone supplementation

Reversible Cause	Typical Symptoms	Diagnosis and Treatment
Vitamin B12 deficiency	Poor concentration, memory loss Generalized weakness, fatigue Abnormal gait, unsteadiness on feet Stomach, gastrointestinal complaints	Physician consultation Tests to evaluate anemia, B12 blood levels, intrinsic factor in the stomach Vitamin B12 injections
Ministrokes	Risk factors of smoking, obesity, high cholesterol, high blood pressure, heart disease, diabetes, family history Sudden or stepwise cognitive decline Fluctuations in course of cognitive decline	Diet: reduce saturated fats, cholesterol Control diabetes, blood pressure Stop smoking Physician consultation CT or MRI scan of the brain Aspirin, ticlopidine, anticoagulants

chug along for years with minimal memory loss induced by a specific, reversible cause like depression or medication toxicity, because it is too subtle to affect daily functioning. Then the process of age-related memory loss, which has been progressing slowly but steadily in the meantime, catches up and adds an extra wallop that leads to clear-cut memory loss. In other words, the two types of memory loss may each be very mild, but when added together, memory loss becomes obvious.

Step 2: Take Sound General Health Measures

General health measures are of great importance in the prevention of age-related memory loss. Diet, exercise, and memory training are the linchpins of these measures to prevent memory loss due to the aging process.

The Essential Promemory Diet
- Decrease intake of saturated fats such as red meat, pizza, desserts.
- Cook with canola, sunflower, corn, or olive oil, which are all high in "good" unsaturated fats.
- Fish has high protein and unsaturated fat content, which lowers the risk of heart attacks and strokes.

- At least two daily helpings each of fruits and vegetables: citrus fruits (oranges, grapefruits; drinking juice instead of eating the actual fruit is okay) and berries are important sources of antioxidants, and green leafy vegetables have essential vitamins.
- Maintain your nonalcohol fluid intake of at least three to five glasses of water daily (more if you do heavy exercise).
- Take a multivitamin tablet daily to boost the promemory effect of a healthy diet. A multivitamin tablet is a supplement, not a substitute, for a healthy diet!
- Supplement with vitamin E, consider taking vitamins A and C as well.

A saturated fat–rich diet is the worst dietary culprit. It can lead to memory loss because high cholesterol levels and plaques begin to block the brain's arteries. Eventually, blood clots can lead to ministrokes and cognitive deficits, depending on which specific part of the brain has been damaged. If hippocampal or frontal cortex nerve cells, or the pathways connecting these regions, are destroyed, memory loss is the result. High levels of saturated fats also generate toxic free radicals, which can damage brain cells even further. Lowering saturated fats boosts the antioxidant potency of your diet, which is beneficial for memory and the aging process more broadly. A diet rich in fresh fruits and vegetables will prevent vitamin deficiencies, promote memory, and reduce the risks of cancer, heart attacks, and stroke.

For further details about the components in the promemory diet, refer back to the table in chapter 5.

Vitamin Supplements Are Good for Your Memory

Diet alone can give you only a moderate amount of promemory antioxidants, and supplementation with vitamins is necessary to boost your antioxidant intake for a promemory effect. I describe the role of antioxidant vitamins E, A, and C, as well as other medications, in your Memory Program later in this chapter.

Aerobic and Anaerobic Exercise

Both aerobic and anaerobic exercise are good for the heart and brain. Aerobic exercise involves medium-level effort in which the heart rate (pulse) rises on average by thirty to forty beats per minute. More severe exertion raises your heart rate even further and takes you into the anaerobic range, which is difficult to keep up for long. As you grow older, there is a good chance that you will shift from mixed anaerobic/ aerobic to pure aerobic activity, tennis to golf. Long walks represent very good aerobic exercise, but with the exception of power walking they do not burn up as many calories as most people think they do.

Exercise Is Important for Your Memory
- Perform moderate, regular exercise three to six times per week.
- Regulate aerobic and anaerobic exercises to your age, health, and tolerance level.
- Aerobic: brisk walking thirty minutes, jogging twenty-five minutes, swimming twenty minutes, formal exercise programs in aerobics classes.
- Mixed aerobic and anaerobic: running, tennis, cycling, exercise equipment (stationary cycle, StairMaster, treadmill, NordicTrack, newer, low-impact workout machines).
- Before you lift weights, start with at least twenty minutes of aerobic or anaerobic cardiovascular fitness exercise (any of the options listed above).
- Yoga and related exercises are excellent for mobility but burn few calories.
- Keep a regular routine: don't overexert one week and become a couch potato the next.
- Stop if breathing difficulty or palpitations or faintness develops.

Regular physical exercise not only improves your general feeling of well-being and quality of life, but it also has a positive impact on memory by decreasing the risk of stroke, releasing endorphins, and possibly stimulating neuronal branching within the brain.

Brain Exercises and Memory Training: Practice Makes Perfect

Exercising the brain can take many forms. It is essential to keep your mind curious, occupied, and creative. Maintaining an active social life as you grow older is crucial, because it is through interaction with other people that your intellect stays sharp. Be mentally active, and cultivate your memory skills to avoid losing them. Several simple strategies, summarized in the table below, can be used to maintain and even boost your memory skills (see more details in chapter 6). Regularity and consistency are necessary for these techniques to have any long-term impact.

Methods to Improve Learning and Recall

Learning New Information	*Recalling Information*
Pay attention.	Go slow if you feel over-whelmed.
Increase sensory and emotional awareness.	Use associations and links.
Focus to register a memory.	Use visual imagery, letters, and rhymes.
Place the event in context.	Chunk numbers and parts of lists.
Consciously repeat it in your mind.	Organize; lists and other memory helpers are essential.
Focus on the gist of what you see or hear.	Trash the junk; create memory storage space.
Above all, be positive about your ability to register new information and to remember it.	

Diet, Physical Exercise, and Memory Training Work Best Together

Obviously, the most effective diet and exercise (physical and mental) program is just that: a diet *and* exercise program, not just one or the other. From a health standpoint, this combination needs to be executed on a steady, continuous basis. Fits and starts are not very helpful in preventing memory loss. Stick to a sensible diet without drastic changes and exercise regularly, preferably a few times each week. Memory training to maintain mental sharpness is also important. Once you convert these changes into regular habits you will be on automatic pilot, and the regimen will not seem so difficult to maintain.

Step 3: Supplement with Medications: Vitamins, Alternative, Pharmaceutical

Medications to prevent future memory loss, or to treat mild forms of memory loss, should be used to supplement, and not replace, general health measures like proper diet and exercise. You may wish to try the alternative medications in the list, or you may prefer to stick to modern pharmaceuticals, which include over-the-counter and prescription medications. But regardless of which camp you belong to, I suggest that you keep an open mind and weigh all the information in your Memory Program before starting any medications.

Individuals React Differently to Different Medications

People react in different ways to the same medications, so if you start with one and you're not happy with it, or feel that you're developing side effects, it is perfectly reasonable to switch to another medication or combination of medications.

Be Realistic: Long-Term Therapy Is Needed to Protect against Memory Loss

You must not forget that a truly effective preventive strategy will take many months to years to exert its full effects, and being impatient about the fact that medications are not giving you a rapid response will be self-defeating. Bear in mind the reality that for age-related memory loss without a specific reversible cause, there is no miracle cure. Blocking further decline, and hopefully experiencing a moderate degree of improvement in memory, should be your goal.

This list of questions to ask your doctor (ask only those questions on the list that are important to you) applies mainly to prescription medications, though it is always a good idea to consult your doctor about over-the-counter and alternative medications as well.

What to Ask Your Doctor about Medications to Improve Memory
- Why am I taking this particular medication?
- How does this medication work on my memory?
- How much improvement can I reasonably expect?
- What is the right dose to take?
- Does it interfere with any other medicines I am taking?
- What are the common side effects?
- How long do I need to take it?
- Is the medicine addictive in any way?
- Can I drink alcohol while taking it?
- Is there any risk in stopping it for a few days at a time?

First-Level Medications

Nonprescription	Prescription
vitamin E	donepezil (Aricept)
phosphatidylserine	estrogen (Premarin)

Second-Level Medications

vitamin A and vitamin C	selegiline (Deprenyl)
aspirin	ginkgo biloba

First-Level Medications: Doses, Actions, Side Effects

My primary or first-level nonprescription choices are vitamin E and phosphatidylserine, with donepezil and estrogen (for women only) making the prescription list.

Vitamin E

Vitamin E's broad antioxidant and antiaging properties vaulted it to the top, particularly as a long-term preventive measure against future memory loss. Vitamin E should be taken as a single daily capsule of 400 to 800 IUs, but you can go up to 1,200 IUs (a maximum of 2,000 IUs if you're very adventurous). There is a very small risk of bleeding if you also take anticoagulants like Coumadin; for the same reason, be cautious about combining vitamin E with aspirin or ginkgo biloba. Fortunately, in the very rare instances of bleeding caused by taking vitamin E, it is likely to begin gradually, so there will be time to reverse the problem by just stopping vitamin E.

A Reminder about Vitamin E
- Vitamin E is present in high-fat foods like vegetable oils, germs, nuts, and seeds.
- It is impossible for you to get more than 200 IUs daily through diet alone.

Phosphatidylserine

Phosphatidylserine is the one medication that has been consistently shown to be superior to placebo in treating age-related memory loss, though all studies have been short-term. It should be taken as 300 mg daily for six to eight weeks followed by 100 mg daily thereafter, based on the notion that a smaller dose is sufficient after the neuronal cell membranes have been saturated with phosphatidylserine. Its lack of side effects, together with its established success in several studies of age-associated memory impairment, helped to get it into the first-level category.

Donepezil (Aricept)

Although donepezil (Aricept) has not been tested in people with mild memory loss, the strength of the data in Alzheimer's disease, which includes FDA approval, as well as clinical experience, led me to elevate it to the A list. You need to be alert to its side effects of nausea and diarrhea, which means that if you are taking another medication that can cause such side effects, such as aspirin, be prepared for stomach discomfort. If this becomes severe, you may need to stop Aricept. Your physician will prescribe Aricept 5 to 10 mg as a single daily dose. Rivastigmine (Exelon) and galantamine (Reminyl) are very similar to Aricept and can substitute for Aricept in the Memory Program.

Estrogen (for Women Only)

Estrogen is only now being directly tested as both a preventive and treatment strategy for mild memory loss due to aging. Even though the results are not yet out, the weight of the evidence supporting its promemory properties is strong. Also, estrogen has broad antiaging properties that include actions against osteoporosis and heart disease, which helped it get top billing. Gynecologic monitoring is essential because of the potential risk of uterine and breast cancer, though using an estrogen-progesterone combination virtually eliminates the increased risk of cancer of the uterus. You need a prescription from your doctor for Premarin 0.625 mg daily (or equivalent), or estrogen-progesterone combinations such as Prempro (over a dozen such combination medications exist).

Second-Level Medications: Doses, Actions, Side Effects

Vitamins A and C

The main reason that vitamins A and C did not make it to the first level is that they have not been rigorously tested against memory loss. Nevertheless, their powerful antioxidant properties, which in animal models have tended to exceed those of vitamin E, suggest potent anti-aging and antimemory loss effects. I also like the fact that they are natural vitamins with few risks attached to their use. Vitamin A supplementation requires 10,000 to 50,000 units daily, or 10,000 to 25,000 units daily when combined with 15 mg beta-carotene. Vitamin C is found in abundance in grapefruits, oranges, and other citrus fruits, but if you wish to try higher doses, take 1 to 5 grams daily in tablet form. Because vitamin C is water soluble, there is no harm in taking even megadoses, because the kidneys can promptly flush them out in the urine. In contrast, megadoses of the fat-soluble vitamins A and E can cause toxicity.

Aspirin

Aspirin's anticoagulant effects help protect against ministrokes, a common cause of memory loss during the aging process. If you have any risk factors for stroke, such as high cholesterol, smoking, or a positive family history of stroke, an aspirin daily (or even a baby aspirin daily) is a good idea. Its anti-inflammatory properties may also be useful in delaying the onset of Alzheimer's disease, and memory loss more generally. Use aspirin with caution if you're prone to stomach upset or irritation (or ulcer), and avoid it if you have bleeding tendencies or are taking anticoagulants.

Ginkgo Biloba

Ginkgo biloba joins phosphatidylserine as an alternative medication that makes the list. EGb 761 is the best-studied form of ginkgo biloba, and can be taken in doses of 120 mg daily. While there is evidence for ginkgo's effectiveness against memory loss, my hesitation in placing it in the first-level category is that the size of its effects against age-related memory loss is very small. Bleeding has been reported when ginkgo is combined with anticoagulant medications; therefore, be cautious about combining it with Vitamin E or aspirin.

Selegiline (Deprenyl)

Selegiline (Deprenyl or Eldepryl) has many actions, including antioxidant properties, that make it an effective antiaging compound. Although its effects in delaying functional deterioration were comparable to those of vitamin E in a recent Alzheimer's study, its use did not lead to improvement in performance on cognitive tests. Like vitamin E, it may be more useful in long-term prevention than it is in treating people who already have memory loss. The recommended dose for this prescription medication is 5 to 15 mg daily.

Why Other Medications Did Not Make the Cut

The cholinergic compounds lecithin and Alcar just missed the cut because the data are much weaker than for Aricept (or Exelon or Reminyl). DHEA (discussed in the next chapter) is not on my list, not only because its efficacy against memory loss has not been established, but also because it is more toxic than the medications that are on the list. The data on hydergine and the nootropics do not suggest sufficient action against memory loss. The COX-II inhibitors did not make it to the list either, mainly because they have just been released and we have no information on their use against memory loss. Ongoing and future clinical studies may demonstrate significant antimemory-loss properties for the COX-II inhibitors, in which case Celebrex or Vioxx might well vault to the top of the list.

The FDA Has Yet to Approve
Any Medication for Mild Memory Loss

Note that none of the prescription medications are approved by the FDA for age-related or mild memory loss, so not all physicians will be willing to prescribe them. However, many neurologists and psychiatrists are prescribing one or more of these medications (off-label) for these purposes.

Long-Term Efficacy Data Are Lacking,
But Safety Data Do Exist

Although I have emphasized that we do not have data about any medications on long-term prevention of memory loss, we do have safety data on long-term use for many of these medications. The vitamins can be taken on a daily basis for years, and so can estrogen in women, provided there is gynecological monitoring. Aricept has been prescribed for several years of continuous usage without major adverse events in Alzheimer's patients, and selegiline has been taken by many Parkinson's patients continuously for several years to decades. Ginkgo biloba also appears to be quite safe during long-term use. Phos-phatidylserine has not been studied in long-term trials, but its lack of side effects during several months of daily administration indirectly suggests that it is likely to be safe even when taken for several years at a stretch.

Which Medications Should You Take?

If you wish to take a memory enhancer, what medication should you choose from this list? Obviously, you cannot take the whole lot for several reasons: the high cost and large number of capsules required, the increased risk of toxicity, and the lack of solid evidence that combinations are better than single agents. Adding selegiline to vitamin E, for example, does not improve matters for patients with Alzheimer's disease, even though individually each agent has a small effect. Critically, combining too many medications can be dangerous because the risk of toxic interactions will skyrocket. The solution is to follow the medication guidelines in the following tables, based on whether you have a normal memory or have mild memory loss.

Medication Regimen to Prevent Memory Loss (Currently Normal Memory)

Medication	Required	Recommended	Optional
Vitamin E	400 to 1,200 IUs daily		
Vitamin C		1 to 5 grams daily	
Vitamin A		10,000 to 25,000 units daily	
Phosphati-dylserine			300 mg daily for 6 to 8 weeks followed by 100 mg daily
Estrogen (post-menopausal women only)		0.625 mg daily (or equivalent)	
Aspirin			325 mg (1 tablet) daily (1 baby aspirin, 81 mg, if adult dose is not tolerated) if you have risk factors for stroke

Medication Regimen to Treat Mild Memory Loss
(without a Reversible Cause)

Medication	Required	Recommended	Optional
Vitamin E	400 to 1,200 IUs daily		
Donepezil (Aricept)		5 to 10 mg daily	
Vitamin C		1 to 5 grams daily	
Vitamin A		10,000 to 25,000 units daily	
Phosphati-dylserine		300 mg daily for 6 to 8 weeks followed by 100 mg daily	
Estrogen (post-menopausal women only)		0.625 mg daily (or equivalent)	
Aspirin		32.5 mg (1 tablet) daily (1 baby aspirin if adult dose not tolerated) if you have risk factors for stroke	
Selegiline (Deprenyl)			5 to 15 mg daily
Ginkgo biloba			120 mg daily (EGb 761)

I will now review the possible combinations of medications, and the Memory Program more broadly, according to categories divided on the basis of age, gender, and preventing future memory loss versus treatment for mild memory loss. I will not repeat the doses and side effects of each medication; this information can be obtained from these tables and the preceding text in this chapter (and earlier chapters).

Customize Your Memory Program

Classify Your Own Memory Status

Place yourself in one of the two categories of normal memory or mild memory loss based on your performance on the tests in the first chapter of this book, and not by relying only on your own subjective view or the opinion of family and friends.

Female, Forty to Fifty-nine Years Old, Currently Normal Memory

- Follow the entire promemory diet (chapter 5 and this chapter).
- Follow the physical exercise regimen (chapter 5 and this chapter), but go easy on running and lifting weights. Equality of the sexes does not extend to bone structure: you need to protect your knees, ankles, and hips more than men of your age. Perform moderate, regular exercise three to six times per week; use any mixture of aerobic and anaerobic exercise that suits your interests.
- Memory exercises and training: this is the right time to begin using all the methods to improve learning and recall that you can use, before memory loss begins to occur.
- Identifying reversible causes of memory loss should not be an issue if you have a normal memory, but it is worth checking the list to see if you have a reversible condition that can be corrected.

Medications

1. Vitamin E 400 to 1,200 IUs daily (400 if you bleed easily, otherwise 800 to 1,200; avoid if taking anticoagulants for medical reasons; do not exceed 400 IUs if you also take aspirin or ginkgo).
2. Consider adding vitamins A and C (see table on page 202) to your diet, which should in any case be rich in these vitamins.
3. If you are worried about future memory loss and want to be very active in preventing it, consider taking phosphatidylserine.
4. If you're postmenopausal, consult your doctor about taking estrogen, both for its promemory and antiosteoporosis effects.
5. Take an aspirin a day if you have risk factors for stroke.

Male, Forty to Fifty-nine Years Old, Currently Normal Memory

- Follow the entire promemory diet (chapter 5 and this chapter).
- Follow the physical exercise regimen (chapter 5 and this chapter): perform moderate, regular exercise three to six times per week; use any mixture of aerobic and anaerobic exercise that suits your interests.

- Memory exercises and training: this is the right time to begin using all the methods to improve learning and recall that you can use, before memory loss begins to occur.
- Identifying reversible causes of memory loss should not be an issue if you have a normal memory, but it is worth checking the list to see if you have a reversible condition that can be corrected.

Medications
1. Vitamin E 400 to 1,200 IUs daily (400 if you bleed easily, otherwise 800 to 1,200; avoid if taking anticoagulants for medical reasons; do not exceed 400 IUs if you also take aspirin or ginkgo).
2. Consider adding vitamins A and C (see table on page 202) to your diet, which should in any case be rich in these vitamins.
3. If you are worried about future memory loss and want to be very active in preventing it, consider taking phosphatidylserine.
4. Take an aspirin a day if you have risk factors for stroke.

Female, Forty to Fifty-nine Years Old, Mild Memory Loss
- Identifying a reversible cause of memory loss should be your top priority; carefully go through the list in this chapter and read the earlier relevant chapters to see if you have a condition worsening your memory. If you think there might be such a cause, or you're not sure, consult your doctor.
- Follow the entire promemory diet (chapter 5 and this chapter).
- Follow the physical exercise regimen (chapter 5 and this chapter), but go easy on running and lifting weights. Equality of the sexes does not extend to bone structure: you need to protect your knees, ankles, and hips more than men of your age. Perform moderate, regular exercise three to six times per week; use any mixture of aerobic and anaerobic exercise that suits your interests.
- Memory exercises and training: try the methods to improve learning and recall that you can use. If you can't do some components, stick to those that you can do without getting too frustrated.

Medications
1. Vitamin E 400 to 1,200 IUs daily (400 if you bleed easily, otherwise 800 to 1,200; avoid if taking anticoagulants for medical reasons; do not exceed 400 IUs if you also take aspirin or ginkgo).

2. Add vitamin A and C supplements (see table on page 203) to your diet, which should already be rich in these vitamins.
3. Consider taking phosphatidylserine as a cognitive enhancer.
4. If you're postmenopausal, consult your doctor about taking estrogen, both for its promemory and antiosteoporosis effects.
5. Talk to your doctor about prescribing donepezil (Aricept; or Exelon or Reminyl), especially if you don't have a clearly identifiable cause of memory loss.
6. You can also ask your doctor about selegiline. Ginkgo biloba is another option. Consider taking only one (or none) of these two medications.
7. Take an aspirin a day if you have risk factors for stroke.

Male, Forty to Fifty-nine Years Old, Mild Memory Loss
- Identifying a reversible cause of memory loss should be your top priority; carefully go through the list in this chapter and read the earlier relevant chapters to see if you have a condition worsening your memory. If you think there might be such a cause, or you're not sure, consult your doctor.
- Follow the entire promemory diet (chapter 5 and this chapter).
- Follow the physical exercise regimen (chapter 5 and this chapter): perform moderate, regular exercise three to six times per week; use any mixture of aerobic and anaerobic exercise that suits your interests.
- Memory exercises and training: try the methods to improve learning and recall that you can use. If you can't do some components, stick to those that you can do without getting too frustrated.

Medications
1. Vitamin E 400 to 1,200 IUs daily (400 if you bleed easily, otherwise 800 to 1,200; avoid if taking anticoagulants for medical reasons; do not exceed 400 IUs if you also take aspirin or ginkgo).
2. Add vitamin A and C supplements (see table on page 203) to your diet, which should already be rich in these vitamins.
3. Consider taking phosphatidylserine as a cognitive enhancer.
4. Talk to your doctor about prescribing donepezil (Aricept; or Exelon or Reminyl), especially if you don't have a clearly identifiable cause of memory loss.

5. You can also ask your doctor about selegiline. Ginkgo biloba is another option. Consider taking only one (or none) of these two medications.
6. Take an aspirin a day if you have risk factors for stroke.

Female, Sixty Years Old or Older, Currently Normal Memory

■ Follow the entire promemory diet (chapter 5 and this chapter).
■ Follow the physical exercise regimen (chapter 5 and this chapter), but go easy on running and lifting weights. Perform moderate, regular exercise three to six times per week, preferably aerobic (e.g., brisk walking or jogging) rather than anaerobic (e.g., running) exercises.
■ Memory exercises and training: it is never too late to begin using the methods to improve learning and recall that you can use. However, you may not achieve as much with these methods as you would have in your forties.
■ Identifying reversible causes of memory loss should not be an issue if you have a normal memory, but it is worth checking the list to see if you have a reversible cause that can be corrected.

Medications

1. Vitamin E 400 to 1,200 IUs daily (400 if you bleed easily, otherwise 800 to 1,200; avoid if taking anticoagulants for medical reasons; do not exceed 400 IUs if you also take aspirin or ginkgo).
2. Consider adding vitamins A and C (see table on page 202) to your diet, which should already be rich in these vitamins.
3. If you are worried about future memory loss and want to be very active in preventing it, consider taking phosphatidylserine.
4. By this age you should have consulted your doctor about taking estrogen, both for its promemory and antiosteoporosis effects.
5. Take an aspirin a day if you have risk factors for stroke.

Male, Sixty Years Old or Older, Currently Normal Memory

■ Follow the entire promemory diet (chapter 5 and this chapter).
■ Follow the physical exercise regimen (chapter 5 and this chapter): perform moderate, regular exercise three to six times per week; preferably aerobic (e.g., brisk walking or jogging) rather than anaerobic (e.g., running) exercises.

- Memory exercises and training: it is never too late to begin using all the methods to improve learning and recall that you can use. However, you may not achieve as much with these methods as you would have in your forties.
- Identifying reversible causes of memory loss should not be an issue if you have a normal memory, but it is worth checking the list in this chapter to see if you have a reversible cause that can be corrected.

Medications
1. Vitamin E 400 to 1,200 IUs daily (400 if you bleed easily, otherwise 800 to 1,200; avoid if taking anticoagulants for medical reasons; do not exceed 400 IUs if you also take aspirin or ginkgo).
2. Consider adding vitamins A and C (see table on page 202) to your diet, which should in any case be rich in these vitamins.
3. If you are worried about future memory loss and want to be very active in preventing it, consider taking phosphatidylserine.
4. Take an aspirin a day if you have risk factors for stroke.

Female, Sixty Years Old or Older, Mild Memory Loss
- Identifying a reversible cause of memory loss should be your top priority; carefully go through the list in this chapter and read the earlier relevant chapters to see if you have a condition worsening your memory. If you think there might be such a cause, or you're not sure, consult your doctor.
- Follow the entire promemory diet (chapter 5 and this chapter).
- Follow the physical exercise regimen (chapter 5 and this chapter), but go easy on running and lifting weights. Equality of the sexes does not extend to bone structure: you need to protect your knees, ankles, and hips more than men of your age. Perform moderate, regular exercise three to six times per week; preferably aerobic over anaerobic exercises.
- Memory exercises and training: try the methods to improve learning and recall that you can use. If you can't do some components, stick to those that you can do without getting too frustrated.

Medications
1. Vitamin E 400 to 1,200 IUs daily (400 if you bleed easily, otherwise 800 to 1,200; avoid if taking anticoagulants for med-

ical reasons; do not exceed 400 IUs if you also take aspirin or ginkgo).

2. Add vitamin A and C supplements (see table on page 203) to your diet, which should already be rich in these vitamins.
3. Consider taking phosphatidylserine as a cognitive enhancer.
4. Talk to your doctor about prescribing donepezil (Aricept; or Exelon or Reminyl), especially if you don't have a clearly identifiable cause of memory loss.
5. You can also ask your doctor about selegiline. Ginkgo biloba is another option. Consider taking only one (or none) of these two medications.
6. Take an aspirin a day if you have risk factors for stroke.

Male, Sixty Years Old or Older, Mild Memory Loss

■ Identifying a reversible cause of memory loss should be your top priority; carefully go through the list in this chapter and read the earlier relevant chapters to see if you have a condition worsening your memory. If you think there might be such a cause, or you're not sure, consult your doctor.
■ Follow the entire promemory diet (chapter 5 and this chapter).
■ Follow the physical exercise regimen (chapter 5 and this chapter): perform moderate, regular exercise three to six times per week; preferably aerobic over anaerobic exercises.
■ Memory exercises and training: try the methods to improve learning and recall that you can use. If you can't do some components, stick to those that you can do without getting too frustrated.

Medications

1. Vitamin E 400 to 1,200 IUs daily (400 if you bleed easily, otherwise 800 to 1,200; avoid if taking anticoagulants for medical reasons; do not exceed 400 IUs if you also take aspirin or ginkgo).
2. Add vitamin A and C supplements (see table on page 203) to your diet, which should already be rich in these vitamins.
3. Consider taking phosphatidylserine as a cognitive enhancer.
4. Talk to your doctor about prescribing donepezil (Aricept; or Exelon or Reminyl), especially if you don't have a clearly identifiable cause of memory loss.
5. You can also ask your doctor about selegiline. Ginkgo biloba is another option. Consider taking only one (or none) of these two medications.
6. Take an aspirin a day if you have risk factors for stroke.

Final Memory Program Tips

1. A combination of general health measures like proper diet and regular exercise, memory training, and appropriate medications (particularly if you have mild memory loss; medications are less critical if you currently have a normal memory), provides a comprehensive strategy to prevent memory loss due to the aging process.

2. If you have mild memory loss, you should first look for a reversible cause.

3. You should feel free to deviate from my recommendations if you have specific health reasons or conditions that make it difficult to implement (medical or other contraindication) one or more of these components in the Memory Program.

4. This field is evolving rapidly, so you need to keep up with the latest developments, which are certain to be given considerable play in the media. These new developments may make it necessary for you to change your strategy over time—for example, you may need to switch to COX-II inhibitors in the future if they are shown to be effective in treating mild memory loss.

CHAPTER 22

Other Potential
Promemory Agents

Many other medications have been proposed as treatments for mild memory loss, or as part of an antiaging regimen. These agents include DHEA, hormones and related peptides, and metallic elements. Although several of these substances are intriguing, the knowledge base is currently insufficient to include them in the Memory Program. Nonetheless, knowing the basic facts will give you a better understanding of the stories that you are likely to hear in the media about one or more of these agents as potential cures for memory loss.

What about DHEA?

Dehydroepiandrosterone, or DHEA, is a natural substance produced primarily by the adrenal glands, which sit on top of the kidneys in the lower back. DHEA is the main starting point for the synthesis of over twenty steroids, including the female hormone estrogen and the male hormone testosterone. Some call it the mother of all steroid hormones.

Actions of DHEA
- Heightens sex drive.
- Raises general activity level.
- Strengthens immune function.

- In mice, maintains neuronal structure, improves the ability to traverse a maze.
- Increases longevity in mice.

In the human brain, DHEA is present at six times its concentration in the bloodstream. In the average person, DHEA blood levels decline fivefold from the age of twenty to seventy years. A few proponents quote this fact to claim that giving DHEA to older people boosts low blood levels and corrects a "deficit." More systematic research is needed to find out if this claim is valid. Of note, in a study of older men, those with the highest DHEA blood levels had the best general health over the course of a decade of follow-up. An alternative to DHEA is pregnenolone, a natural steroid that is converted to DHEA in the body.

DHEA: Clinical Impact on Memory

Clinically, some patients with lupus who take DHEA have reported improved mood and less generalized pain. DHEA has also been administered to people with a variety of age-related maladies, including memory loss. A major limitation is that most studies to date have involved only a handful of subjects. German investigators recently reported that a single 300 mg dose of DHEA did not affect memory test performance in young adults. In another negative study, Kristine Yaffe, in San Francisco, found no associations between DHEA blood levels and cognitive test performance in a community sample of 394 women. On the other hand, a small uncontrolled study conducted within the NIH in Bethesda, Maryland, suggests that DHEA can treat memory loss in patients with dementia. But until the acid test of a large-scale, double-blind, placebo-controlled trial has been passed, the jury will still be out on this compound.

DHEA Side Effects Can Be Serious

DHEA's conversion to steroid hormones underlies some of its therapeutic effects, but the same properties can lead to toxicity. DHEA raises the levels of testosterone and other male hormones, which increases the risk of prostate cancer. I strongly recommend medical evaluation and clearance by a physician, including assessment of blood prostate-specific antigen (PSA), for any middle-aged or elderly man who chooses to embark on DHEA therapy.

Another side effect is an increase in masculine features such as growth of facial hair and acne. As a result, DHEA is rarely given to women, who also risk losing scalp hair and developing a bass voice. Proper medical monitoring is essential. Daily doses of DHEA cover a range from 25 to 200 mg daily, with an average of 50 mg daily. This range is wide because some physicians adjust the dose to maintain high blood levels of DHEA, a scientifically unproven practice.

Hormone and Peptide Therapy

If thyroid deficiency causes memory loss, can giving thyroid hormone to people without this hormone deficiency boost memory? The answer is no: the body's internal regulatory system maintains a fine balance in the levels of thyroid and most other hormones, quickly getting rid of the excess hormone that is ingested. An additional factor weighing against these hormones is that they cause a variety of side effects (differs markedly among different hormones) when given in high doses, thus reducing their potential utility as a long-term preventive strategy against age-related memory loss.

Vasopressin, also called antidiuretic hormone, is produced by cells that lie just above the pituitary gland in the brain. Studies in mice indicate that vasopressin improves learning and memory, but clinical results have been disappointing. Vasopressin is difficult to use because it needs to be given intravenously or via a nasal spray, and its effects on blood pressure and the kidneys make it potentially dangerous when used in high doses.

Other hormones, and some peptides that are similar to hormones, have each been proposed as potential antimemory-loss agents, but no scientific basis has been found for these claims. These include melanotropin, atrial natriuretic peptide, and substance P.

Metallic Elements Are Present in Trace Quantities

Metallic elements like chromium, magnesium, and selenium are essential elements that are normally ingested only in trace quantities. These elements hold some promise in the fight against memory loss.

Selenium

Selenium is an integral part of the enzyme glutathione peroxidase, which protects cell membranes. Selenium is a strong antioxidant, and therefore may work against memory loss, but this has not been tested systematically. The daily dietary requirement of selenium is 70 micrograms for men and 55 micrograms for women, and is easily obtained from grains, nuts, fish, and dairy products.

Magnesium

Both magnesium and selenium increase the production of antibodies and enhance immune system function. Magnesium is also a catalyst for enzymes involved in energy production, and helps to regulate cell membrane stability. This range of actions has lent it some standing as an antiaging and antimemory-loss therapy, but systematic clinical studies have not yet been conducted.

Magnesium may have antianxiety and antistress properties. Since magnesium has cardiac effects, if you are a heart patient you need to check with your doctor if you plan to start taking magnesium supplements. Magnesium is chemically very similar to calcium, and the two have to be in close balance—yin and yang—for proper bodily function. Therefore, high calcium intake needs to accompany magnesium therapy. Magnesium is present in a variety of foodstuffs: fruits, dairy products, green leafy vegetables, whole grains, nuts, and seafood. A normal diet easily exceeds the FDA minimum daily requirement of 350 mg for men and 280 mg for women.

Aluminum

Metals like chromium, magnesium, and selenium compete with aluminum in some of their actions because they occupy similar positions in the periodic table of natural elements. The interest in these elements accelerated after the aluminum theory of Alzheimer's disease was proposed. In the early 1980s, traces of aluminum were found in the plaques and tangles that develop in the brains of patients with Alzheimer's disease. However, community surveys across the world show no link between aluminum exposure and dementia, or even milder forms of memory loss. As a result, research in this area has floundered in recent years. Few studies have been conducted with any of these metals as a treatment for memory loss.

Chromium

Chromium is essential in the manufacture of trypsin, an important digestive enzyme in the intestines. Chromium is also present in red blood cells and helps to metabolize cholesterol, thereby reducing the risk of atherosclerosis. Most diets are sufficient in chromium, except for elderly people with poor diets. Supplements are available as chromium picolinate, but should not be taken in excess because of the risk of toxicity. Although on a theoretical basis chromium may have promemory properties, there are no worthwhile research data on this issue.

Boron

Boron is another metallic element that acts in the brain. It improves electrical activity in nerve cells and seems to speed up reaction time and general alertness. It is also necessary for the body to properly process calcium, magnesium, and phosphorus. Fruits and nuts have a high boron content. Since only a minuscule dietary intake is necessary, deficiency of this element is extremely rare. There are no clinical studies showing an effect against memory loss.

Zinc

Antiaging Properties of Zinc
- Helps to heal wounds and repair skin damage.
- Facilitates the action of antioxidants like vitamin E.
- Increases the efficiency of the immune system.
- Present in high concentrations in the hippocampus.
- Involved either as a catalyst or in the chemical structure of over three hundred enzymes.
- Levels decline with age, and some practitioners recommend zinc supplements as part of an antiaging program.

Zinc's utility against memory loss remains to be tested clinically. In an elegant series of laboratory experiments in animals, Dennis Choi, chairman of the department of neurology at Washington University in St. Louis, showed that zinc in low concentrations protects against some types of hippocampal neuronal injury, but that at higher concentrations it kills nerve cells. So zinc therapy may be a double-edged sword: at low doses it is good, at high doses it is bad. This twist has led to a reversal in therapeutic strategies for memory loss; zinc therapy is now being replaced by substances that actually decrease zinc's availability in the brain. Zinc is present in concentrations that are sometimes too low to detect, but new technology has opened up opportunities that should eventually tell us a great deal about the functions of zinc and all the other metallic trace elements in the brain.

The FDA recommended daily requirement for zinc is 15 mg for men and 12 mg for women, and this is easily obtained through a wide range of foods. Rarely, elderly people who suffer from general malnutrition can develop zinc deficiency, for which the main symptom is lack of taste and poor appetite. In high doses, zinc can cause stomach irritation, so if you plan to use zinc supplements, do so in moderation.

Iron

What about iron, one of the most common metals in your body? Iron is an essential component of hemoglobin, which is a big molecule inside red blood cells that carries oxygen throughout the body, including the brain. Iron deficiency can lead to anemia, which in severe cases can cause weakness, fatigue, and secondary cognitive impairment. The treatment is iron replacement (tablets). In the absence of iron deficiency, taking iron supplements will not boost your memory. I do not recommend iron supplementation in the absence of anemia, because excessive iron intake can damage the liver and other internal organs, as well as predispose you to a heart attack.

Trace Elements: To Take or Not To Take Them

Except for iron, all the heavy metals described in this section come under the category of "trace" elements because they are needed in microscopic quantities for normal bodily function. These metals can become toxic if taken in high doses. You may recall my earlier story about how my father's Parkinson's disease was going to be treated with an Ayurvedic heavy metal concoction, and I put a stop to it because of the potential for toxicity. Traces of lead, mercury, or arsenic, which are indistinguishable to the naked eye when mixed with other metals, can be extremely dangerous and even fatal. Therefore, if you plan to take a metallic supplement of any type, you must buy it from a reputed manufacturing source, preferably one with a national or international reputation.

As you've noticed, none of the trace metals made it into the Memory Program, largely because of the lack of systematic controlled studies with any of them.

CHAPTER 23

Your Future Memory Program

THE LONG-STANDING DEFEATISM about preventing and treating memory loss has now given way to a feeling of growing excitement that we will soon have the keys to the memory kingdom. But we have just scratched the surface, and new knowledge will eventually render obsolete our current repertoire of preventive and treatment strategies, including some of the components in the Memory Program.

Several potential therapies for age-related memory loss are still in the development stage. These include a new crop of cholinesterase inhibitors, treatment with combinations of cognitive enhancers, stimulation of neuronal growth, blocking the formation of toxic compounds in the brain, and genetic strategies. Most of these attempts are likely to fail, but the few gems that emerge will revolutionize the field of memory loss research and potentially could completely reverse the memory loss that occurs during the aging process.

Cholinesterase Inhibitors

Cholinesterase inhibitors represent the only class of medications that are FDA-approved to treat dementia, specifically Alzheimer's disease. After tacrine came donepezil (Aricept), rivastigmine (Exelon), and galantamine (Reminyl). Although these medications were developed to treat patients with Alzheimer's disease, the pharmaceutical industry has become aware that the market for mild memory loss is much larger.

217

Aricept has been shown to improve cognition in patients with multiple sclerosis, and is now being tested in people with mild to moderate memory loss. The other newer cholinergic agents may have similar properties. The underlying rationale is that cholinergic nerve cells decay in all of us during the aging process, and cholinesterase inhibitors can reverse this deficit and thereby improve cognitive performance.

Combination Therapies Need to Be Tested

From a theoretical perspective, tackling different pathways that lead to memory loss may be more beneficial than dealing with only one pathway, but a few studies that attempted combination therapies met with poor results. The Alzheimer's study using vitamin E plus selegiline showed no advantage for the combination over either medication taken alone. Earlier, Ken Davis's group at Mount Sinai Medical Center in New York tried a medication cocktail to simultaneously correct the cholinergic and adrenergic (norepinephrine) deficits in Alzheimer's disease, but the combination did not work well in a clinical trial.

But another incidental finding suggests that the search for an optimal combination therapy should not be abandoned. In the tacrine study of patients with Alzheimer's disease, the medication's effect was strongest in women taking estrogen, indicating that the combination was better than tacrine alone. In an entirely different field, AIDS treatment underwent a revolution after combinations of protease inhibitors were shown to be much more effective than single medication regimens. In the future, I expect that a number of combinations will be studied from the potpourri of therapies for memory loss: ginkgo biloba, donepezil, vitamin E, estrogen, and COX-II inhibitors, to name a few. At this stage, it is impossible to predict which combination of two or three or four medications will prove superior to treatment with individual medications.

Note that the Memory Program relies on a multilayered strategy that includes the judicious use of carefully selected combinations of medications.

Stimulating Nerve Cell Growth

In infant mice, an enriched environment of toys, high-quality food, games, and other stimuli increases nerve cell growth and branching in the brain. Compared to normally caged mice living a spartan existence, mice exposed to barely two months of this enriched environment show a 15 percent increase in the number of brain nerve cells. You know that in children, intensive education accompanied by strong nurturing and healthy social stimulation often leads to outstanding academic and subsequent professional success. It is as if these environmental factors are the cognitive enhancers, the promemory agents, of childhood. But can a similar approach be used to boost memory in older people, whose nerve cells have largely lost the ability to reproduce?

Substances that stimulate the growth and branching of existing nerve cells, without necessarily increasing their number through a reproductive process, may enhance cognitive abilities. For example, infusing a naturally occurring substance called nerve growth factor into mice increases neuronal branching and improves connectivity among brain cells. These ideas are still in animal experimentation, but clinical trials are likely to begin with one or more neurotrophic compounds in the near future.

Pluripotent Nerve Cells: A Neuroscience Controversy

A healthy diet, regular exercise, and intellectual and social stimulation are clearly beneficial to brain function. There is a molecular basis to the effects of these types of environmental stimulation in the brain. Although most nerve cells in an older person's brain have indeed lost the ability to reproduce, there are a few primitive cells, called pluripotent cells, that retain the capacity to differentiate or evolve into several types of nerve cells at any time during the life span, including old age. While these cells are small in number, they can still play an important restorative role after injury or damage or the aging process itself. Some of these pluripotent neural cells appear to be present in the hippocampus, and stimulating them to differentiate and reproduce may prove to be an excellent promemory strategy. As a matter of fact, a few drug companies are trying to develop neurotrophic compounds that can stimulate these primitive, pluripotent cells to differentiate and grow into functioning nerve cells in the brain.

Basic research on pluripotent nerve cells has been very limited, and some scientists question if they even exist in the adult human brain.

Transplantation

A more direct human application is transplantation, which has been tried with dopamine-producing cells in Parkinson's patients who suffer from dopamine deficiency. In the early work, human fetal cells that produced dopamine were transplanted, because such cells are more likely to retain the capacity to reproduce than adult cells. Later, the abortion controversy led to a U.S. ban on the use of fetal tissue in medical research or procedures. This political detour submerged the revolutionary impact of the finding that cells from outside the body can actually survive and reproduce after being placed inside the brain. A Mexican neurosurgeon reported the initial successful transplants in Parkinson's disease, but Scandinavian and American doctors could not replicate the results, and the jury is still out on this issue. But note that long-term follow-up of these transplanted Parkinson's patients has revealed a disturbing side effect: involuntary jerks and movements caused by the transplanted dopamine cells continuing to reproduce, because the normal regulatory mechanisms that suppress their action within the brain don't work well on transplanted cells.

Memory loss involves the hippocampus and surrounding areas, which are relatively small regions, but also the frontal cortex, which occupies a huge portion of the brain's surface. This wide representation of memory in the brain makes transplantation an unlikely candidate for the next memory "cure." Nonetheless, if a method can be developed to transplant cells that reproduce and differentiate into hippocampal nerve cells, preferably cholinergic nerve cells, the field would truly be revolutionized. My prediction, however, is that highly effective promemory medications will be developed long before implantation of cells into the brain can be used to solve the problem of memory loss.

Blocking Formation of Toxic Compounds

Most of the existing therapies, and those in research development, focus on stimulating natural promemory factors—the good guys—in the brain, or by blocking destruction of the good guys (e.g., cholinesterase inhibitors). But what about the opposite strategy: blocking the bad guys—the toxic enzymes, the destructive genes and neurotransmitters that trigger and mediate cell death? Antioxidants represent one such approach. But in recent years, the focus has shifted to more sophisticated techniques that attempt to block the formation of deposits in the brain that damage nerve cells. These deposits, which are called amyloid plaques and neurofibrillary tangles, typically occur in Alzheimer's disease. The same plaques are present, though to a much lesser extent, in elderly people with age-related memory loss. So the question naturally arises: what if we could block the formation of plaques and tangles in the first place?

Preventing Amyloid Formation

Many drug companies are now in hot pursuit of compounds (Beta-block is the name of one such drug in development) that can block the enzymes that trigger the formation of Beta-amyloid, which is the main protein component of the amyloid plaque. Recently, an experimental vaccine has also been developed for this purpose. Many of these compounds are toxic, and we are still a long way from translating these concepts into a clinically useful treatment. But if it does occur, millions of patients and families with dementia, particularly Alzheimer's disease, will be eternally grateful.

Blocking Neurotransmitters

There may be ways to either block the formation or increase the destruction of other naturally occurring toxic chemicals and neurotransmitters, which include nitric oxide, n-methyl-d-aspartate (NMDA), and glutamate. Studies with glutamate antagonists have been unsuccessful in clinical trials of patients with dementia, and fiddling with NMDA receptor function can be dangerous because of the risk of seizures. Part of the problem is that we currently do not have a complete understanding of how exactly these chemicals and neurotransmitters work in the brain, and what impact they have on memory processes. As research evolves, compounds that can better target the right neurotransmitter sites within the brain will be developed.

Genetic Strategies: There Is No "Memory Gene"

The more we learn about the brain, the more it becomes clear that there is no single "memory gene" that holds the key. A complex web of interacting genes, chemicals, and neurotransmitters is involved in an intricate dance to keep our brains ticking along accurately, and at the right pace.

Genetics is the holy grail of new technology in medicine. There is a lot of hype, which reaches a crescendo with every breakthrough, be it the cloning of sheep or a new treatment for breast cancer. But in my view, the hype is justified. An incredible number of diseases are primarily genetic in origin, and we have little to no idea as to how to treat them, except for therapies that treat the symptoms but not the disease itself. As our knowledge about human genetic structure and function grows, more and more genetically engineered treatments will emerge. Eventually, some of our science fiction fantasies will be transformed into human reality.

A large part of the human genome, or genetic map, focuses on controlling protein synthesis within the brain. As of now, we do not know which genes are responsible for triggering the process of neuronal degeneration and death in the hippocampus and frontal lobes, or for that matter any other part of the brain. It is likely that we all possess both "good memory genes" and "bad memory genes," and once we discover them we will be able to directly tackle the problem of age-related memory loss that affects most of us as we grow older.

CREB and Knockout Mice

A memory trace is solidified if there is a small gap in time between the pieces of information that need to be remembered. Using this technique, which is called spaced training, scientists engineered a fruit fly to have a photographic memory. In the same fruit fly species, they triggered a master gene called CREB, which has the ability to goad a number of other genes into action. In this manner, the fruit fly with a fabulous memory was born. Ideally, if we could stimulate CREB in the same way in the human brain, total recall would become the standard for everyone. But there is no known method to turn a gene on or off in the human brain, so even though we all possess CREB, we don't yet know how to galvanize it into action in people. The goal of these researchers is to see if manipulating CREB in some fashion will make it possible to unlock the full power of human memory.

Other researchers like Eric Kandel approach the same problem from a different angle. He takes mice and removes, or knocks out, a gene or set of genes that are involved in cognitive processes. These "knockout" mice perform horribly in mazes and similar tests of cognitive ability. Drugs are then administered, one by one, to see if they can reverse this glaring memory deficit in the knockout mice. One such promising agent is rolipram, but as yet there are no worthwhile clinical studies with this compound. Another strategy is to block the synthesis of specific proteins by genetic manipulation, which then leads to memory loss in rats. As with the knockout mice, specific drugs can be given to reverse this process and correct the memory deficit. Kandel, in his dynamic way, has formed his own company to employ these techniques to try and find the magic pill that will reverse memory loss.

Other Novel Strategies

AMPA receptors are present throughout the brain, and are involved in synaptic connections between brain cells. These AMPA receptors play a role in boosting both learning and memory, and ampakines are substances that amplify or enhance these signals. Some investigators are trying to develop drugs that can amplify the AMPA signal, while others believe that this is a waste of time because ampakines share many similarities to caffeine, which improves attention and mental arousal with no direct impact on memory.

In animal models, a number of other substances can amplify long-term potentiation, which is the physiologic property of cells to remain depolarized, or stimulated, for an extended period of time. Kandel and other researchers believe that at the cellular level, long-term potentiation is the method by which a memory trace becomes solidified and is eventually transferred into long-term memory storage. A number of chemicals can amplify the effects of long-term potentiation. These include substances that stimulate dopamine receptors and others that inhibit the enzyme phosphodiesterase. In animal studies, these chemical substances improve transfer of information from short- to long-term storage. But as of yet, there are no clinical studies to back up these intriguing laboratory findings.

Earlier, I referred to Dennis Choi's work on zinc and memory. Although few other researchers are putting much time and energy into studying metallic elements that are known to be involved in essential enzyme pathways, my guess is that this will change in the future. Sophisticated new technologies will help us to decipher what exactly these trace metals like chromium and selenium are doing in the brain. Future therapies may be based on increasing or decreasing the levels of these metallic elements in a targeted fashion, taking into account the delicate balance that exists between these metallic elements and a variety of processes in the brain.

The elusive prion, discovered by Nobel laureate Stanley Prusiner, must not be forgotten. These microscopic prions play a role not only in neurological disorders, but possibly in memory loss due to the aging process itself. I suspect that we will hear a lot more about the role of prions in memory loss.

A Bright Future Awaits

The graveyard of memory research has turned into a fertile field budding with roses of all shapes and colors. The rose isn't a bad analogy;

while the final product will be extremely beautiful, you are likely to meet a few thorns along the way. In this book, I have reviewed our current knowledge base and laid out a comprehensive program to help you prevent memory loss due to the aging process, or to identify and treat mild memory loss if it has already set in. But all this is based on current knowledge, which is clearly limited in many ways. Given the various research directions that the field is taking, what does the future hold?

Research in molecular genetics, neuroscience, and clinical trials is growing at a blinding pace and is likely to accelerate. Part of this pressure comes from the worldwide exponential increase in knowledge, and part of it comes from you. You comprise the largest segment of the population with the most political clout, and at least when it comes to funding medical research, the politicians are responding.

If things pan out the way that some experts hope, every Kodak moment will literally be inside your head in a perfect image, and cameras will become obsolete. But I do not entirely subscribe to this view, because the fact is that human memory is finite. We all have to wipe out old, useless memories to make way for the new, important ones. We do this daily, as our hippocampi and frontal lobes deliberately forget what we ate for lunch yesterday, two days ago, a week ago, and so forth. Therefore, at least for the foreseeable future, I expect that new treatments will be able to completely block memory loss, but they will not be able to give us total recall. Total recall would mean cluttering up our brains with sundry, often worthless information, and life would become impossible to manage.

Larger societal questions will spring forth as memory enhancement becomes a universal tool. Will people in high-precision jobs that do not permit error, such as highfliers on Wall Street or surgeons in the operating room, be required to take memory enhancers as a matter of course? And the courts, which are already nightmarish in their complexity—what will they do about witnesses who do or don't take promemory agents? And what about the opposite end of the age spectrum: will children be made to take memory enhancers to perform well in school the way they now use computers and the Internet to boost academic performance?

These possibilities lie well into the future. For now, I urge you to begin, and then maintain, the Memory Program to prevent memory loss, and to directly tackle mild memory loss if it has already begun to affect your life. I predict that as time goes on, you are likely to look back with satisfaction at the results that you have achieved.

BIBLIOGRAPHY

Alexander, G. E., Furey, M. L., Grady, C. L., Pietrini, P., Brady, D. R., Mentis, M. J., Schapiro, M. B. Association of premorbid intellectual function with cerebral metabolism in Alzheimer's disease: implications for the cognitive reserve hypothesis. *American Journal of Psychiatry* 154:165–172, 1997.

Alexopoulos, G. S., Meyers, B. S., Young, R. C., Mattis, S., Kakuma, T. The course of geriatric depression with "reversible dementia": a controlled study. *American Journal of Psychiatry* 150:1693–1699, 1993.

Amaducci, L., and the Smid group. Phosphatidylserine in the treatment of Alzheimer's disease: results of multicenter study. *Psychopharmacology Bulletin* 24:130–134, 1988.

Amaducci, L. A., Fratiglioni, L., Rocca, W. A., et al. Risk factors for clinically diagnosed Alzheimer's disease: a case-control study of Italian population. *Neurology* 36:922–931, 1986.

Anschutz, L., Camp, C., Markley, R., Kramer, J. Remembering mnemonics: A three-year follow-up on the effects of mnemonics training in elderly adults. *Experimental Aging Research* 13:141–143, 1987.

Argyriou, A., Prast, H., Philippu, A. Melatonin facilitates short-term memory. *European Journal of Pharmacology* 349:159–162, 1998.

Backman, L., Small, B. J. Influences of cognitive support on episodic remembering: tracing the process of loss from normal aging to Alzheimer's disease. *Psychology and Aging* 13:267–276, 1998.

Ball, M. J., Hachinski, V., Fox, A., et al. A new definition of Alzheimer's disease: a hippocampal dementia. *Lancet* 5:14–16, 1985.

Barber, R., Scheltens, P., Gholkar, A., Ballard, C., McKeith, I., Ince, P., Perry, R., O'Brien, J. White matter lesions on magnetic resonance imaging in dementia with Lewy bodies, Alzheimer's disease, vascular dementia, and normal aging. *Journal of Neurology, Neurosurgery and Psychiatry* 67:66–72, 1999.

Barona, A., Reynolds, C., Chastain, R. A demographically based index of permorbid intelligence for the WAIS-R. *Journal of Consulting and Clinical Psychology* 52:885–887, 1984.

Bartzokis, G., Beckson, M., Hance, D. B., Po, H., Foster, J. A., Mintz, J., Ling, W., Bridge, P. Magnetic resonance imaging evidence of "silent" cerebrovascular toxicity in cocaine dependence. *Biological Psychiatry* 45:1203–1211, 1999.

Bechara, A., Tranel, D., Damasio, H., Adolphs, R., Rockland, C., Damasio, A. R. Double dissociation of conditioning and declarative knowledge relative to the amygdala and hippocampus in humans. *Science* 269:1115–1118, 1995.

225

Berg, L., McKeel, D. W., Miller, J. P., Storandt, M., Rubin, E. H., Morris, J. C., Baty, J., et al. Clinicopathologic studies in cognitively healthy aging and Alzheimer disease. *Archives of Neurology* 55:326–330, 1998.

Berr, C., Lafont, S., Debuire, B., Dartigues, J. F., Baulieu, E. E. Relationships of dehydroepiandrosterone sulfate (DHEA) in the elderly with functional, psychological and mental status, and short-term mortality: a French community-based study. *Proceedings of the National Academy of Sciences, USA* 93:13410–13415, 1996.

Block, R. I., Wittenborn, J. R. Marijuana effects on the speed of memory retrieval in the letter-matching task. *International Journal of the Addictions* 21:281–285, 1986.

Bowen, J. D., Larson, E. B. Drug-induced cognitive impairment: defining the problem and finding solutions. *Drugs and Aging* 3:349–357, 1993.

Buschke, H., Fuld, P. A. Evaluating storage, retention, and retrieval in disordered memory and learning. *Neurology* 24:1019–1025, 1974.

Buschke, H., Kuslansky, G., Katz, M., Stewart, W. F., Silwinski, M. J., Eckholdt, H. M., Lipton, R. B. Screening for dementia with the memory impairment screen. *Neurology* 52:231–238, 1999.

Caffarra, P., Santamaria, V. The effects of phosphatidylserine in patients with mild cognitive decline. *Clinical Trials Journal* 24:109–114, 1987.

Cassone, M. C., Molinengo, L. Action of thyroid hormones, diazepam, caffeine, and amitriptyline on memory decay ("forgetting"). *Life Sciences* 29:1983–1988, 1981.

Cavanaugh, J. C., Grady, J. G., Perlmutter, M. Forgetting and use of memory aids in 20- to 70-year olds' everyday life. *International Journal of Aging and Human Development* 17:113–122, 1983.

Chandra, V., Kokmen, E., Schoenberg, B. S., Beard, C. M. Head trauma with loss of consciousness as a risk factor for Alzheimer's disease. *Neurology* 39:1576–1578, 1989.

Choi, D. W., Koh, J. Y. Zinc and brain injury. *Annual Review of Neuroscience* 21:347–375, 1998.

Christensen, H., Korten, A., Jorm, A. F., Henderson, A. S., Scott, R., MacKinnon, A. J. Activity levels and cognitive functioning in an elderly community sample. *Age and Aging* 25:72–80, 1996.

Christianson, S. A., Loftus, E. F. Memory for traumatic events. *Applied Cognitive Psychology* 1:225–233, 1987.

Claus, J. J., van Harskamp, F., Breteler, M. M. B., Krenning, E. P., de Koning, I., van der Cammen, T. J. M., Hofman, A., et al. The diagnostic value of SPECT with Tc 99m HMPAO in Alzheimer's disease: a population-based study. *Neurology* 44:454–461, 1994.

Coria, F., Gomez de Caso, J. A., Minguez, L., Rodriguez-Artalejo, F., Claveria, L. E. Prevalence of age-associated memory impairment and dementia in a rural community. *Journal of Neurology, Neurosurgery and Psychiatry* 56:973–976, 1993.

Corkin, S. Functional MRI for studying episodic memory in aging and Alzheimer's disease. *Geriatrics* 53(Suppl 1):S13–15, 1998.

Costa, M. M., Reus, V. I., Wolkowitz, O. M., Manfredi, F., Lieberman, M. Estrogen replacement therapy and cognitive decline in memory-impaired postmenopausal women. *Biological Psychiatry* 46:182–188, 1999.

Cowley, C., Underwood, A. Memory. *Newsweek*, pages 49–52. June 15, 1998.

Crook, T. H., Adderley, B. *The Memory Cure.* Pocket Books, New York, 1998.

Crook, T. H., Tinklenberg, J., Yesavage, J., Petrie, W., Nunzi, M. G., Massari, D. C. Effects of phosphatidylserine in age-associated memory impairment. *Neurology* 41:644–649, 1991.

Damasio, A. R. Consciousness. Knowing how, knowing where. *Nature* 375:106–107, 1995.

Damasio, H., Grabowski, T. J., Tranel, D., Hichwa, R. D., Damasio, A. R. A neural basis for lexical retrieval. *Nature* 380:499–505, 1996.

Davies, G., Alonso-Quecuty, M. Cultural factors in the recall of a witnessed event. *Memory* 5:601–614, 1997.

de la Monte, S. M., Ghanbari, K., Frey, W. H., Beheshti, I., Averback, P., Hauser, S. L., Ghanbari, H. A., et al. Characterization of the AD7C-NTP cDNA expression in Alzheimer's disease and measurement of a 41-kD protein in cerebrospinal fluid. *Journal of Clinical Investigation* 100:3093–3104, 1997.

de Leon, M. J., Convit, A., DeSanti, S., Bobinski, M., George, A. E., Wisniewski, H. M., Rusinek, H., et al. Contribution of structural neuroimaging to the early diagnosis of Alzheimer's disease. *International Psychogeriatrics* 9:183–190, 1997.

Devanand, D. P., Folz, M., Gorlyn, M., Moeller, J. R., Stern, Y. Questionable dementia: course and predictors of outcome. *Journal of the American Geriatric Society* 45:321–328, 1997.

Devanand, D. P., Sano, M., Tang, M. X., Taylor, S., Gurland, B. J., Wilder, D., Stern, Y., et al. Depressed mood and the incidence of Alzheimer's disease in the elderly living in the community. *Archives of General Psychiatry* 53:175–182, 1996.

Devanand, D. P., Michaels-Marston, K. S., Liu, X., Pelton, G. H., Padilla, M., Marder, K., Bell, K., Stern, Y., Mayeux, R. Olfactory deficits in patients with mild cognitive impairment predict Alzheimer's disease at follow-up. *American Journal of Psychiatry* 157:1399–1405, 2000.

DeWeer, B., Lehericy, S., Pillon, B., Baulac, M., Chiras, J., Marsault, C., Agid, Y., et al. Memory disorders in probable Alzheimer's disease: the role of hippocampal atrophy as shown with MRI. *Journal of Neurology, Neurosurgery and Psychiatry* 58:590–597, 1995.

Di Luca, M., Pastorino, L., Bianchetti, A., Perez, J., Vignolo, L. A., Lenzi, G. L., Trabucchi, M., Cattabeni, F., Padovani, A. Differential level of platelet amyloid beta precursor protein isoforms: an early marker for Alzheimer disease. *Archives of Neurology* 55:1195–2000, 1998.

Doraiswamy, P. M., Steffens, D. C. Combination therapy for Alzheimer's disease: what are we waiting for? *Journal of the American Geriatrics Society* 46:1322–1324, 1998.

Doty, R. L., Reyes, P. F., Gregor, T. Presence of both odor identification and detection deficits in Alzheimer's disease. *Brain Research Bulletin* 18:597–600, 1987.

Enns, M., Peeling, J., Sutherland, G. R. Hippocampal nerve cells are damaged by caffeine-augmented electroshock seizures. *Biological Psychiatry* 40:642–647, 1996.

Erber, J. T., Szuchman, L. T., Rothberg, S. T. Dimensions of self-report about everyday memory in young and older adults. *International Journal of Aging and Human Development* 34:311–323, 1992.

Evans, D. A., Hebert, L. E., Beckett, L. A., Scherr, P. A., Albert, M. S., Chown, M. J., Pilgrim, D. M., et al. Education and other measures of socioeconomic status and risk of incident Alzheimer disease in a defined population of older persons. *Archives of Neurology* 54:1399–1405, 1997.

Farlow, M., Gracon, S. I., Hershey, L. A., Lewis, K. W., Sadowsky, C. H., Dolan-Ureno, J., for the Tacrine Study Group. *Journal of the American Medical Association* 268:2523–2529, 1992.

Fiatarone, M. A., O'Neill, E. F., Ryan, N. D., Clements, K. M., Solares, G. R., Nelson, M. E., Roberts, S. B., Kehayias, J. J., Lipsitz, L. A., Evans, W. J. Exercise training and nutritional supplementation for physical frailty in very elderly people. *New England Journal of Medicine* 330:1769–1775, 1994.

FitzSimon, J. S., Waring, S. C., Kokmen, E., McLaren, J. W., Brubaker, R. F. Response of the pupil to tropicamide is not a reliable test for Alzheimer disease. *Archives of Neurology* 54:155–159, 1997.

Folstein, M., Folstein, S., McHugh, P. "Mini-mental state": a practical method of grading the cognitive state of patients for clinicians. *Journal of Psychiatric Research* 12:189–198, 1975.

Forbes, W. F., Lessard, S., Gentleman, J. F. Geochemical risk factors for mental functioning, based on the Ontario longitudinal study of aging (LSA) V. comparisons of the results, relevant to aluminium water concentrations, obtained from the LSA and from death certificates mentioning dementia. *Canadian Journal on Aging* 14:642–646, 1995.

Foster, R. G. Shedding light on the biological clock. *Neuron* 20:829–832, 1998.

Fox, N. C., Warrington, E. K., Seiffer, A. L., Agnew, S. K., Rossor, M. N. Presymptomatic cognitive deficits in individuals at risk of familial Alzheimer's disease. A longitudinal prospective study. *Brain* 121:1631–1639, 1998.

Fuld, P. A., Masur, D. M., Blau, A. D., Crystal, H., Aronson, M. K. Object-memory evaluation for prospective detection of dementia in normal functioning elderly: predictive and normative data. *Journal of Clinical and Experimental Neuropsychology* 12:520–528, 1990.

Gagnon, M., Letenneur, L., Dartigues, J. F., Commenges, D., Orgogozo, J. M., Gateau, P. B., Alperovitch, A., et al. Validity of the mini-mental state examination as a screening instrument for cognitive impairment and dementia in French elderly community residents. *Neuroepidemiology* 9:143–150, 1990.

Galasko, D., Clark, C., Chang, L., Miller, B., et al. Assessment of CSF levels of tau protein in mildly demented patients with Alzheimer's disease. *Neurology* 48:632–635, 1997.

Gao, S., Hendrie, H. C., Hall, K. S., Hui, S. The relationships between age, sex, and the incidence of dementia and Alzheimer disease: a meta-analysis. *Archives of General Psychiatry* 55:809–815, 1998.

Ghanbari, H., Ghanbari, K., Beheshti, I., Munzar, M., Vasauskas, A., Averback, P. Biochemical assay for AD7C-NTP in urine as an Alzheimer's disease marker. *Journal of Clinical and Laboratory Analysis* 12:285–288, 1998.

Gilewski, M. J., Zelinski, E. M., Schaie, K. W. The Memory Functioning Questionnaire for the assessment of memory complaints in adulthood and old age. *Psychology and Aging* 5:482–490, 1990.

Giovagnoli, A. R., Mascheroni, S., Avanzini, G. Self-reporting of everyday memory in patients with epilepsy: relation to neuropsychological, clinical, pathological and treatment factors. *Epilepsy Research* 28:119–128, 1997.

Golomb, J., Kluger, A., de Leon, M. J., Ferris, S. H., Mittelman, M., Cohen, J., George, A. E. Hippocampal formation size predicts declining memory performance in normal aging. *Neurology* 47:810–813, 1996.

Gould, E. C., Woolley, C. S., McEwen, B. S. The hippocampal formation: morphological changes induced by thyroid, gonadal, and adrenal hormones. *Psychoneuroendocrinology* 16:67–84, 1991.

Gower, T. Is there a magic memory bullet? *Esquire,* page 142, December 1997.

Grant, S., London, E., Newlin, D. B., Villemagne, V. L., Liu, X., Contoreggi, C., Phillips, R. L., Kimes, A. S., Margolin, A. Activation of memory circuits during cue-elicited cocaine craving. *Proceedings of the National Academy of Sciences* 93:12040–12045, 1996.

Greenwood, C. E., Winocur, G. Learning and memory impairment in rats fed a high saturated fat diet. *Behavioral Neurology and Biology* 53:74–87, 1990.

Growdon, J. H., Graefe, K., Tenis, M., Hayden, D., Schoenfeld, D., Wray, S. H. Pupil dilation to tropicamide is not specific for Alzheimer disease. *Archives of Neurology* 54:841–844, 1997.

Hall, S. S. Our memories, our selves. *New York Times Sunday Magazine*, pages 26–33, 49–57. February 15, 1998.

Hanninen, M. A., Hallikainen, M., Koivisto, K., et al. A follow-up study of age-associated memory impairment: neuropsychological predictors of dementia. *Journal of the American Geriatric Society* 43:1007–1015, 1995.

Hassing, L., Wahlin, A., Winblad, B., Backman, L. Further evidence on the effects of vitamin B12 and folate levels on episodic memory functioning: a population-based study of healthy very old adults. *Biological Psychiatry* 45:1472–1480, 1999.

Hayaishi, O. Tryptophan, oxygen, and sleep. *Annual Review of Biochemistry* 63:1–24, 1994.

Heishman, S. J., Arasteh, K., Stitzer, M. L. Comparative effects of alcohol and marijuana on mood, memory, and performance. *Pharmacology and Biochemistry of Behavior* 58:93–101, 1997.

Hendler, N., Cimini, C., Ma, T., Long, D. A comparison of cognitive impairment due to benzodiazepines and to narcotics. *American Journal of Psychiatry* 137:828–830, 1980.

Heseker, H., Schneider, R. Requirement and supply of vitamin C, E and beta-carotene for elderly men and women. *European Journal of Clinical Nutrition* 48:118–127, 1994.

Heyman, A., Fillenbaum, G. G., Welsh-Bohmer, K. A., Gearing, M., Mirra, S. S., Mohs, R. C., Peterson, R. L., Pieper, C. F. Cerebral infarcts with autopsy-proven Alzheimer's disease: CERAD, part XVIII. Consortium to Establish a Registry for Alzheimer's Disease. *Neurology* 51:159–162, 1998.

Higbee, K. L. *Your Memory: How It Works and How to Improve It*, Second edition. Paragon House, New York, 1988.

Hyman, S. T., Gomaz-Isla, T., Briggs, M., Chung, H., Nichols, S., Kohout, F., Wallace, R. Apolipoprotein E and cognitive change in an elderly population. *Annals of Neurology* 40:55–66, 1996.

Israel, L., Melac, M., Milinkevitch, D., Dubos, G. Drug therapy and memory training programs: a double-blind randomized trial of general practice patients with age-associated memory impairment. *International Psychogeriatrics* 6:155–170, 1994.

Jabs, T. Reactive oxygen intermediates as mediators of programmed cell death in plants and animals. *Biochemical Pharmacology* 57:231–245, 1999.

Jack, C. R. Jr., Petersen, R. C., Xu, Y., O'Brien, P. C., Smith, G. E., Ivnik, R. J., Tangalos, E. G., Kokmen, E. Rate of medial temporal lobe atrophy in typical aging and Alzheimer's disease. *Neurology* 51:993–999, 1998.

Jacobs, D. M., Sano, M., Dooneief, G., Marder, K., Bell, K. L., Stern, Y. Neuropsychological detection and characterization of preclinical Alzheimer's disease. *Neurology* 45:957–962, 1995.

Jacobsen F.M., Comas-Diaz L. Donepezil for psychotropic-induced memory loss. *Journal of Clinical Psychiatry* 60:698–704, 1999.

Jama, J. W., Launer, L. J., Witteman, J. C., den Breeijen, J. H., Breteler, M. M., Grobbee, D. E., Hofman, A. Dietary antioxidants and cognitive function in a population-based sample of older persons. The Rotterdam study. *American Journal of Epidemiology* 144:275–280, 1996.

Jazwinski, M. J. Longevity, genes, and aging. *Science* 273:54–58, 1996.

Jimenez-Jimenez, F. J., Molina, J. A., de Bustos, F., Orti-Pareja, M., Benito-Leon, J., Tallon-Barranco, A., Gasalla, T., Porta, J., Arenas, J. Serum levels of beta-carotene, alpha-carotene and vitamin A in patients with Alzheimer's disease. *European Journal of Neurology* 6:495–497, 1999.

Johansson, B., Zarit, S. H. Early cognitive markers of the incidence of dementia and mortality: a longitudinal population-based study of the oldest old. *International Journal of Geriatric Psychiatry* 12:53–59, 1997.

Jonker, C., Launer, L. J., Hooijer, C., Lindeboom, J. Memory complaints and memory impairment in older individuals. *Journal of the American Geriatrics Society* 44:44–49, 1996.

Kandel, E. R. Genes, synapses, and long-term memory. *Journal of Cell Physiology* 173:124–125, 1997.

Kandel, E. R., Abel, T. Neuropeptides, adenyl cyclase, and memory storage. *Science* 268:825–826, 1995.

Kawas, C. S., Resnick, S., Morrison, A., Brookmeyer, R., Corrada, M., Zonderman, A., Bacal, C., Lingle, D. D., Metter, E. A prospective study of estrogen replacement therapy and the risk of developing Alzheimer's disease: the Baltimore longitudinal study of aging. *Neurology* 48:1517–1521, 1997.

Keller, M. B., McCullough, J. P., Klein, D. N., Arnow, B., Dunner, D. L., Gelenberg, A. J., Markowitz, J. C., Nemeroff, C. B., Russell, J. M., Thase, M. E., Trivedi, M. H., Zajecka, J. A comparison of nefazodone, the cognitive behavioral-analysis system of psychotherapy, and their combination for the treatment of chronic depression. *New England Journal of Medicine* 342:1462–1470, 2000.

Kliegl, R., Smith, J., Baltes, P. B. Testing-the-limits and the study of adult age differences in cognitive plasticity of a mnemonic skill. *Developmental Psychology* 25:247–256, 1989.

Koivisto, K., Reinikainen, K. J., Vanhanen, M., Helkala, E., Mykkannen, L., Laakso, M., Pyorala, K., et al. Prevalence of age-associated memory impairment in a randomly selected population from eastern Finland. *Neurology* 45:741–747, 1995.

Kral, V. A. Senescent forgetfulness, benign and malignant. *Canadian Medical Association Journal* 86:257–260, 1962.

Kramer, A. F., Hahn, S., Cohen, N. J., Banich, M. T., McAuley, E., Harrison, C. R., Chason, J., Vakil, E., Bardell, L., Boileau, R. A., Colcombe, A. Ageing, fitness and neurocognitive function. *Nature* 400:418–419, 1999.

Lang, F. R., Carstensen, L. L. Close emotional relationships in late life: further support for proactive aging in the social domain. *Psychological Aging* 9:315–324, 1994.

Launer, L. J., Masaki, K., Petrovitch, H., Foley, D., Havlik, R. J. The association between midlife blood pressure levels and late-life cognitive function. The Honolulu Asia aging study. *Journal of the American Medical Association* 274:1846–1851, 1995.

Le Bars, P. L., Katz, M. M., Berman, N., Itil, T. M., Freedman, A. M., Schatzberg, A. F. A placebo-controlled, double-blind, randomized trial of an extract of ginkgo biloba for dementia. *Journal of the American Medical Association* 278:1327–1332, 1997.

Lemonick, M. D. Beyond depression. What do these "mood drugs" really do? *Time* 153:74, May 17, 1999.

Leo, M. A., Lieber, C. S. Alcohol, vitamin A, and beta-carotene: adverse interactions, including hepatotoxicity and carcinogenicity. American Journal of Clinical Nutrition 69:1071–1085, 1999.

Letzel, H., Haan, J., Feil, W. B. Nootropics: efficacy and tolerability of products from three active substance classes. *Journal of Drug Decision in Clinical Practice* 8:77–94, 1996.

Lipsky, P. E. The clinical potential of cyclooxygenase-2 inhibitors. *American Journal of Medicine* 106(5B):51S–57S, 1999.

Lissner, L., Bengtsson, C., Bjorkelund, C., Wedel, H. Physical activity levels and changes in relation to longevity. A prospective study of Swedish women. *American Journal of Epidemiology* 143:54–62, 1996.

Loke, W. H. Effects of caffeine on mood and memory. *Physiology and Behavior* 44:367–372, 1988.

Lucca, U., Tettamanti, M., Forloni, G., Spagnoli, A. Nonsteroidal anti-inflammatory drug use in Alzheimer's disease. *Biological Psychiatry* 36:854–856, 1994.

Lund-Manchester Group. Clinical and neuropathological criteria for frontotemporal dementia. *Journal of Neurology, Neurosurgery and Psychiatry* 57:416–418, 1994.

Martzke, J. S., Kopala, L. C., Good, K. C. Olfactory disfunction in neuropsychiatric disorders: review and methodological considerations. *Biological Psychiatry* 42:721–732, 1997.

Marwick, C. Growing use of medicinal botanicals forces assessment by drug regulators. *Journal of the American Medical Association* 273:607–609, 1995.

Masuda, Y., Kokubu, T., Yamashita, M., Ikeda, H., Inoue, S. Egg phosphatidylcholine combined with vitamin B12 improved memory impairment following lesioning of nucleus basalis in rats. *Life Sciences* 62:813–822, 1998.

Matthews, M. K. Association of ginkgo biloba with intracerebral hemorrhage. *Neurology* (letter) 50:1933–1934, 1998.

Mayeux, R., Saunders, A. M., Shea, S., Mirra, S., Evans, D., Roses, A., Hyman, B., et al. Utility of the apolipoprotein e genotype in the diagnosis of Alzheimer's disease. *New England Journal of Medicine* 338:506–511, 1998.

Maylor, E. A., Rabbitt, P. M. Effect of alcohol on rate of forgetting. *Psychopharmacology* (Berlin) 91:230–235, 1987.

McCleary, R., Dick, M. B., Buckwalter, G., Henderson, V. Full-information models for multiple psychometric tests: annualized rates of change in normal aging and dementia. *Alzheimer Disease and Associated Disorders* 10:216–223, 1996.

McEwen, B. S. Permanence of brain sex differences and structural plasticity of the adult brain. *Proceedings of the National Academy of Sciences* 96:7128–7130, 1999.

―――. Protective and damaging effects of stress mediators. *New England Journal of Medicine* 338:171–179, 1998.

―――. Stress and hippocampal plasticity. *Annual Review of Neuroscience* 22:105–122, 1999.

McEwen, B. S., Alves, S. E. Estrogen actions in the central nervous system. *Endocrinology Review* 20:279–307, 1999.

McGeer, P. L., Schulzer, M., McGeer, E. G. Arthritis and anti-inflammatory agents as possible protective factors for Alzheimer's disease: a review of 17 epidemiologic studies. *Neurology* 47:425–432, 1996.

McKeith, I. G., Galasko, D., Kosaka, K., Perry, E. K., Dickson, D. W., Hansen, L. A., Salmon, D. P., et al. Consensus guidelines for the clinical and pathologic diagnosis of dementia with Lewy bodies (DLB): report of the consortium on DLB international workshop. *Neurology* 47:1113–1124, 1996.

Means, L. W., Higgins, J. L., Fernandez, T. J. Mid-life onset of dietary restriction extends life and prolongs cognitive functioning. *Physiology and Behavior* 54:503–508, 1993.

Meier, B. Industry's next growth sector: memory lapses. *New York Times,* pages 1, 17, April 4, 1999.

Mendelsohn, A. B., Belle, S. H., Stoehr, G. P., Ganguli, M. Use of antioxidant supplements and its association with cognitive function in a rural elderly cohort: the MoVIES project. Monongahela Valley Independent Elders Survey. *American Journal of Epidemiology* 148:38–44, 1998.

Miller, G. A. The magical number seven: plus or minus two. Some limits on our capacity for processing information. *Psychological Review* 9:81–97, 1956.

Mohs, R. C., Ashman, T. A., Jantzen, K., Albert, M., Brandt, J., Gordon, B., Rasmusson, X., Grossman, M., Jacobs, D., Stern, Y. A study of the efficacy of a comprehensive memory enhancement program in healthy elderly persons. *Psychiatry Research* 77:183–195, 1998.

Morris, J. C., Storandt, M., McKeel, D. W., Rubin, E. H., Price, J. L., Grant, E. A., Berg, L. Cerebral amyloid deposition and diffuse plaques in "normal" aging: evidence for presymptomatic and very mild Alzheimer's disease. *Neurology* 46:707–719, 1996.

Mulnard, R. A., Cotman, C. W., Kawas, C., van Dyck, C. H., Sano, M., Doody, R., Koss, E., Pfeiffer, E., Jin, S., Gamst, A., Grundman, M., Thomas, R., Thal, L. J. Estrogen replacement therapy for treatment of mild to moderate Alzheimer disease: a randomized controlled trial. Alzheimer's Disease Cooperative Study. *Journal of the American Medical Association* 283:1007–15, 2000.

Newcomer, J. W., Selke, G., Melson, A. K., Hershey, T., Craft, S., Richards, K., Alderson, A. L. Decreased memory performance in healthy humans induced by stress-level cortisol treatment. *Archives of General Psychiatry* 56:527–533, 1999.

Newman, P. E. Could diet be used to reduce the risk of Alzheimer's disease? *Medical Hypotheses* 50:335–337, 1998.

Nordin, S., Murphy, C. Odor memory in normal aging and Alzheimer's disease. *Annals of the New York Academy of Sciences* 855:686–693, 1998.

Oken, B. S., Storzbach, D. M., Kaye, J. A. The efficacy of ginkgo biloba on cognitive function in Alzheimer disease. *Archives of Neurology* 55:1409–1415, 1998.

Orentreich, N., Brind, J. L. Long-term longitudinal measurements of plasma dehydroepiandrosterone sulfate in normal men. *Journal of Clinical Endocrinology and Metabolism* 75:1002–1004, 1992.

Osterweil, D., Syndulko, K., Cohen, N., Pettler-Jennings, P. D., Hershman, J. M., Cummings, J. L., Tourtellotte, W. W., Solomon, D. H. Cognitive function in nondemented older adults with hypothyroidism. *Journal of the American Geriatric Society* 40:325–335, 1992.

Perrig, W. J., Perrig, P., Stahelin, H. B. The relation between antioxidants and memory performance in the old and very old. *Journal of the American Geriatrics Society* 45:718–724, 1997.

Petersen, R. C. Normal aging, mild cognitive impairment, and early Alzheimer's disease. *The Neurologist* 1:326–344, 1995.

Peterson, R. C., Smith, G. E., Waring, S. C., Ivnik, R. J., Tangalos, E. G., Kokmen, E. Mild cognitive impairment: clinical characterization and outcome. *Archives of Neurology* 56:303–308, 1999.

Plassman, B. L., Welsh, K. A., Helms, M., Brandt, J., Page, W. F., Breitner, J. C. Intelligence and education as predictors of cognitive state in late life: a 50-year follow-up. *Neurology* 45:1446–1450, 1995.

Rai, G. S., Shovlin, C., Wesnes, K. A. A double-blind placebo-controlled study of ginkgo biloba extract ("Tanakan") in elderly outpatients with mild to moderate memory impairment. *Current Medical Research Opinion* 12:350–355, 1991.

Reid, L. D., Johnson, R. E., Gettman, D. A. Benzodiazepine exposure and functional status in older people. *Journal of the American Geriatric Society* 46:71–76, 1998.

Reisberg, B., Ferris, S. H., Anand, R., Mir, P., Geibel, V., De Leon, M. J. Effects of naloxone in senile dementia: a double-blind trial. *New England Journal of Medicine* 308:721–722, 1983.

Reisberg, B., Ferris, S. H., Franssen, E., Kluger, A., Borenstein, J. Age-associated memory impairment: the clinical syndrome. *Developmental Neuropsychology* 2:401–412, 1986.

Rogers, S. L., Farlow, M. R., Doody, R. S., Mohs, R., Friedhoff, L. T., and the Donepezil study group. A 24-week, double-blind, placebo-controlled trial of donepezil in patients with Alzheimer's disease. *Neurology* 50:136–145, 1998.

Rosler, M., Anand, R., Cicin-Sain, A., Gauthier, S., Agid, Y., Dal-Bianco, P., Stahelin, H. B., Hartman, R., Gharabawi, M. Efficacy and safety of rivastigmine in patients with Alzheimer's disease: international randomised controlled trial. *British Medical Journal* 318(7184):633–638, 1999.

Ryabinin, A. E. Role of hippocampus in alcohol-induced memory impairment: implications from behavioral and early gene studies. *Psychopharmacology* 139:34–43, 1998.

Sackeim, H. A., Steif, B. L. The neuropsychology of depression and mania. In: Georgotas, A., Cancro, R., eds. *Depression and Mania*. New York: Elsevier, 1988:265–289.

Sano, M., Ernesto, C., Thomas, R. G., Klauber, M. R. A controlled trial of selegiline, alpha-tocopherol, or both as treatment for Alzheimer's disease. *New England Journal of Medicine* 336:1216–1222, 1997.

Sapolsky, R. M., Krey, L. C., McEwen, B. S. The neuroendocrinology of stress and aging: the glucocorticoid cascade hypothesis. *Endocrinology Review* 7:284–301, 1986.

Satoh, T., Sakurai, I., Miyagi, K., Hohsaku, Y. Walking exercise and improved neuropsychological functioning in elderly patients with cardiac disease. *Journal of Internal Medicine* 238:423–428, 1995.

Schacter, D. L. *Searching for memory: the brain, the mind, and the past.* Basic Books, New York, 1996.

Schenk, D., Barbour, R., Dunn, W., Gordon, G., Grajeda, H., Guido, T., Hu, K., Huang, J., Johnson-Wood, K., Khan, K., Kholodenko, D., Lee, M., Liao, Z., Lieberburg, I., Motter, R., Mutter, L., Soriano, F., Shopp, G., Vasquez, N., Vandevert, C., Walker, S., Wogulis, M., Yednock, T., Games, D., Seubert, P. Immunization with amyloid-beta attenuates Alzheimer-disease-like pathology in the PDAPP mouse. *Nature* 400:173–177, 1999.

Schmand, B., Jonker, C., Hooijer, C., Lindeboom, J. Subjective memory complaints may announce dementia. *Neurology* 46:121–125, 1996.

Scogin, F., Bienias, J. A three-year follow-up of older adult participants in a memory skills training program. *Psychology and Aging* 3:334–337, 1988.

Shapiro, S. L., Schwartz, G. E., Bonner, G. Effects of mindfulness-based stress reduction on medical and premedical students. *Journal of Behavioral Medicine* 21:581–599, 1998.

Slaven, L., Lee, C. Mood and symptom reporting among middle-aged women: the relationship between menopausal status, hormone replacement therapy, and exercise participation. *Health Psychology* 16:203–208, 1997.

Slotten, H. A., Krekling, S. Does melatonin have an effect on cognitive performance? *Psychoneuroendocrinology* 21:673–680, 1996.

Small, G. W., La Rue, A., Komo, S., Kaplan, A., Mandelkern, M. A. Predictors of cognitive change in middle-aged and older adults with memory loss. *American Journal of Psychiatry* 152:1757–1764, 1995.

Snowdon, D. A., Griener, L. H., Mortimer, J. A., Riley, K. P., Greiner, P. A., Markesbery, W. R. Brain infarction and the clinical expression of Alzheimer's disease: the nun study. *Journal of the American Medical Association* 277:813–817, 1997.

Snowdon, D. A., Kemper, S. J., Mortimer, J. A., Greiner, L. H., Wekstein, D. R., Markesbery, W. R. Linguistic ability in early life and cognitive function and Alzheimer's disease in late life. Findings from the nuns study. *Journal of the American Medical Association* 275:528–532, 1996.

Socci, D. J., Crandall, B. M., Arendash, G. W. Chronic antioxidant treatment improves the cognitive performance of aged rats. *Brain Research* 693:88–94, 1995.

Solfrizzi, V., Panza, F., Torres, F., Mastroianni, F., Del Parigi, A., Venezia, A., Capurso, A. High monounsaturated fatty acids intake protects against age-related cognitive decline. *Neurology* 52:1563–1569, 1999.

Solomon, P. R., Hirschoff, A., Kelly, B., Relin, M., Brush, M., DeVeaux, R. D., Pendlebury, W. W. A 7-minute neurocognitive screening battery highly sensitive to Alzheimer's disease. *Archives of Neurology* 55:349–355, 1998.

Stern, Y., Gurland, B., Tatemichi, T. K., Tang, M. X., Wilder, D., Mayeux, R. Influence of education and occupation on the incidence of Alzheimer's disease. *Journal of the American Medical Association* 271:1004–1010, 1994.

Stern, Y., Sano, M., Mayeux, R. Long-term administration of oral physostigmine in Alzheimer's disease. *Neurology* 38:1837–1841, 1988.

Stoll, S., Hafner, U., Pohl, W. E., Muller, W. E. Age-related memory decline and longevity under treatment with selegiline. *Life Sciences* 55:2155–2163, 1994.

Suhr, J., Tranel, D., Wefel, J., Barrash, J. Memory performance after head injury: contributions of malingering, litigation status, psychological factors, and medication use. *Journal of Clinical and Experimental Neuropsychology* 19:500–514, 1997.

Summers, W. K., Majovski, L. V., Marsh, G. M., Tachiki, K., Kling, A. Oral tetrahydroaminoacridine in long-term treatment of senile dementia, Alzheimer type. *New England Journal of Medicine* 315:1241–1245, 1986.

Sunderland, A., Stewart, F. M., Sluman, S. M. Adaptation to cognitive deficit? An exploration of apparent dissociations between everyday memory and test performance late after stroke. *British Journal of Clinical Psychology* 35:463–476, 1996.

Tang, M. X., Jacobs, D., Stern, Y., Marder, K., Schofield, P., Gurland, B., Andrews, H., Mayeux, R. Effect of oestrogen during menopause on risk and age at onset of Alzheimer's disease. *Lancet* 348:429–432, 1996.

Tariot, P. N., Solomon, P. R., Morris, J. C., Kershaw, P., Lilienfeld, S., Ding, C. A 5-month, randomized, placebo-controlled trial of galantamine in AD. The Galantamine USA-10 Study Group. *Neurology* 54:2269–2276, 2000.

Thal, L. J., Carta, A., Clarke, W. R., Ferris, S. H., Friedland, R. P., Peterson, R. C., Pettegrew, J. W., Pfeiffer, E., Raskind, M. A., Sano, M., Tuszynski, M. H., Woolson, R. F. A 1-year multicenter placebo-controlled study of acetyl-l-carnitine in patients with Alzheimer's disease. *Neurology* 47:705–711, 1996.

Tierney, M. C., Szalai, J. P., Snow, W. G., Fisher, R. H., Tsuda, T., Chi, H., McLachlan, D. R., St. George-Hyslop, P. H. A prospective study of the clinical utility of ApoE genotype in the prediction of outcome in patients with memory impairment. *Neurology* 46:149–154, 1996.

Tierney, M. C., Szalai, J. P., Snow, W. G., Fisher, R. H., Nores, A., Nadon, G., Dunn, E., et al. Prediction of probable Alzheimer's disease in memory-impaired patients: a prospective longitudinal study. *Neurology* 46:661–665, 1996.

Tracy, J. I., Bates, M. E. The selective effects of alcohol on automatic and effortful memory processes. *Neuropsychology* 13:282–290, 1999.

Trojanowski, J. Q., Growdon, J. H. A new consensus report on biomarkers for the early antemortem diagnosis of Alzheimer disease: current status, relevance to drug discovery, and recommendations for future research (editorial). *Journal of Neuropathology and Experimental Neurology* 57:643–644, 1998.

Tune, L., Carr, S., Hoag, E., Cooper, T. Anticholinergic effects of drugs commonly prescribed for the elderly: potential means for assessing risk of delirium. *American Journal of Psychiatry* 149:1393–1394, 1992.

Van Gijn, J. Low doses of aspirin in stroke prevention. *Lancet* 353:2172–2173, 1999.

Van Gorp, W. G., Wilkins, J. N., Moore, L. H., Hull, J., Horner, M. D., Plotkin, D. Declarative and procedural memory functioning in abstinent cocaine abusers. *Archives of General Psychiatry* 56:85–89, 1999.

Van Ryn, J., Pairet, M. Clinical experience with cyclooxygenase-2 inhibitors. *Inflammation Research* 48:247–254, 1999.

Verhaeghen, P., Marcoen, A., Goossens, L. Facts and fiction about memory aging: a quantitative integration of research findings. *Journal of Gerontology* 48:157–171, 1993.

Vernon, M. W., Sorkin, E. M. Piracetam. An overview of its pharmacological properties and a review of its therapeutic use in senile cognitive disorders. *Drugs and Aging* 1:17–35, 1991.

Warburton, D. M. Effects of caffeine on cognition and mood without caffeine abstinence. *Psychopharmacology* (Berlin) 119:66–70, 1995.

Watkins, P. B., Zimmerman, H. J., Knapp, M. J., Gracon, S. I., Lewis, K. W. Hepatotoxic effects of tacrine administration in patients with Alzheimer's disease. *Journal of the American Medical Association* 271:992–998, 1994.

West, R. L., Crook, T. H., Barron, K. L. Everyday memory performance across the life span: effects of age and noncognitive individual differences. *Psychology and Aging* 7:72–82, 1992.

Wolf, O. T., Neumann, O., Hellhammer, D. H., Geiben, A. C., Strassburger, C. J., Dressendorfer, R. A., et al. Effects of a two-week physiological DHEA substitution on cognitive performance and well-being in healthy elderly women and men. *Journal of Endocrinological Investigation* 82:2363–2367, 1997.

Woodle, E. S., Kulkarni, S. Programmed cell death. *Transplantation* 66:681–691, 1998.

Yaffe, K., Ettinger, B., Pressman, A., Seeley, D., Whooley, M., Schaefer, C., Cummings, S. Neuropsychiatric function and dehydroepiandrosterone sulfate in elderly women: a prospective study. *Biological Psychiatry* 43:694–700, 1998.

Yaffe, K., Sawaya, G., Lieberburg, I., Grady, D. Estrogen therapy in postmenopausal women: effects on cognitive function and dementia. *Journal of the American Medical Association* 279:688–695, 1998.

Young, E. A. DHEA: Mood, memory, and aging. *Biological Psychiatry* 45:1531–1532, 1999.

Zola-Morgan, S. M., Squire, L. R. The primate hippocampal formation: evidence for a time-limited role in memory storage. *Science* 250:288–290, 1990.

RESOURCES

Alzheimer's Association
919 N. Michigan Ave, #1000
Chicago IL 60611-1676
800-272-3900
www.alz.org

Alzheimer's Disease (Memory Disorders) Centers

These centers are funded by the National Institute of Aging (part of the NIH)and focus on research and clinical services for patients with Alzheimer's disease (www.alzheimers.org), but in recent years they have expanded their efforts to patients with mild to moderate memory loss. If you suffer from mild to moderate memory loss, and wish to seek expert physician consultation, it is worth going to a center that is in your geographic region. The clinicians and researchers in these centers (the name and telephone number of the director of each center, as of mid-2000, are listed below) are the leading experts in the field of memory disorders.

Lindy E. Harrell, M.D., Ph.D.
Professor, Department of Neurology
University of Alabama at Birmingham
1720 Seventh Avenue South
Birmingham, AL 35294-0017
Tel: 205-934-2178

William J. Jagust, M.D.
Director, UC Davis Alzheimer's Disease
  Center
150 Muir Road (127A)
Martinez, CA 94553
Tel: 510-372-2485

Jeffrey L. Cummings, M.D.
Professor of Neurology and Psychiatry
UCLA Medical Center
710 Westwood Plaza
Los Angeles, CA 90095-1769
Tel: 310-206-5238

Leon Thal, M.D.
Chairman, Department of Neuroscience
U.C. San Diego School of Medicine
9500 Gilman Drive
La Jolla, CA 92093-0624
Tel: 619-622-5800

Caleb E. Finch, Ph.D.
Ethel Percy Andrus Gerontology Center
University Park, MC-0191
3715 McClintock Avenue
Los Angeles, CA 90089-0191
Tel: 213-740-7777

Mahlon E. Delong, M.D.
Emory Alzheimer's Disease Center
Wesley Woods Health Center
1841 Clifton Road NE
Atlanta, GA 30329
Tel: 404-728-6950

237

Marsel Mesulam, M.D.
Director, Alzheimer's Center
Northwestern University Medical School
320 East Superior Street, Searle 11-450
Chicago, IL 60611
Tel: 312-908-9339

Denis E. Evans, M.D.
Rush-Presbyterian Alzheimer's Disease
  Center
1645 West Jackson Boulevard, Suite 675
Chicago, IL 60612
Tel: 312-942-4463

Bernardino Ghetti, M.D.
Indiana Alzheimer's Disease Center
635 Barnhill Drive
Indianapolis, IN 46202-5120
Tel: 317-278-2030

Charles DeCarli, M.D.
Department of Neurology
University of Kansas Medical Center
3901 Rainbow Boulevard, G043
Kansas City, KS 66160-7314
Tel: 913-588-6979

William R. Markesbery, M.D.
Sanders-Brown Research Center on
  Aging
University of Kentucky
101 Sanders-Brown Building
800 South Lime
Lexington, KY 40536-0230
Tel: 606-323-6040

Donald L. Price, M.D.
Johns Hopkins University
558 Ross Research Building
720 Rutland Avenue
Baltimore, MD 21205-2196
Tel: 410-955-5632

Neil William Kowall, M.D.
Alzheimer's Disease Center, Boston University
Bedford VA Medical Center (182B)
200 Springs Road
Bedford, MA 01730
Tel: 781-687-2916

John H. Growdon, M.D.
Massachusetts Alzheimer's Disease
  Research Center
Massachusetts General Hospital, WAC 830
15 Parkman Street
Boston, MA 02114
Tel: 617-726-1728

Sid Gilman, M.D.
Michigan Alzheimer's Disease Research
  Center
University of Michigan
1914 Taubman Center
Ann Arbor, MI 48109-0316
Tel: 313-764-2190

Ronald C. Petersen, M.D., Ph.D.,
Professor of Neurology, Mayo Clinic
200 First Street SW
Rochester, MN 55905
Tel: 507-284-1324

Eugene M. Johnson Jr., Ph.D.
Alzheimer's Disease Research Center
Washington University School of Medicine
4488 Forest Park Avenue, Suite 130
St. Louis, MO 63108-2293
Tel: 314-286-2881

Michael L. Shelanski, M.D., Ph.D.
Columbia University
630 West 168th Street
New York, NY 10032
Tel: 212-543-5853

Kenneth L. Davis, M.D.
Mount Sinai School of Medicine
One Gustave L. Levy Place, Box 1230
New York, NY 10029-6574
Tel: 212-241-8329

INDEX

ABOUT THE AUTHOR

D. P. Devanand, M.D., who completed his specialty training at Yale University School of Medicine, is professor of clinical psychiatry and neurology at the College of Physicians and Surgeons of Columbia University, New York, where he is codirector of the Memory Disorders Center. A practicing physician, he is board-certified with added subspecialty certification in geriatric psychiatry. He is the principal investigator of several research grants from the National Institutes of Health and private foundations. He has published two books and over 130 research and clinical articles and book chapters. Dr. Devanand currently resides in New York City.